The Menopause and HRT

The publishers wish to draw your attention to the following error on page 94:

- The doses of **ESTRADERM MX** should be 25mcg, 50mcg, 100mcg.
- The doses of **EVOREL** should be 25mcg, 50 mcg, <u>75mcg</u>, 100mcg.

The following products to be included in the table:

Unopposed oestrogen - Elleste Solo 1mg, 2mg

Sequential combined - Elleste Duet 2mg (containing norethisterone), Femapak 40mcg (containing Dydrogesterone), Prempak C 0.625 mg, 1.25mg (containing norgestrel)

The Menopause and HRT

Kathy Abernethy

Clinical Nurse Specialist (Menopause)
Northwick Park Hospital
Harrow, Middlesex

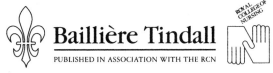

Baillière Tindall
PUBLISHED IN ASSOCIATION WITH THE RCN

London   Philadelphia   Toronto   Sydney   Tokyo

Baillière Tindall   24–28 Oval Road
London NW1 7DX

The Curtis Center
Independence Square West
Philadelphia, PA 19106-3399, USA

Harcourt Brace & Company
55 Horner Avenue
Toronto, Ontario, M8Z 4X6, Canada

Harcourt Brace & Company, Australia
30–52 Smidmore Street
Marrickville
NSW 2204, Australia

Harcourt Brace & Company, Japan
Ichibancho Central Building
Chiyoda-ku, Tokyo 102, Japan

A catalogue record for this book is available from the British
Library

ISBN 0-7020-2023-0

Typeset by Paston Press Ltd, Loddon, Norfolk
Printed and bound in Great Britain by WBC, Bridgend,
Mid Glamorgan

Contents

Chapter 1

What is the Menopause?

We have all heard and read about 'the menopause' but
the term is one which is often used to mean different
things to different people. To some women it is simply an
explanation of a physiological change taking place in
their bodies. To others, the word itself triggers negative
thoughts about middle age and loss of femininity. Most
women will recognize that the time of the menopause is a
time of hormonal disturbance, but many will not understand precisely what those changes are or what causes
them to happen. This chapter will help you understand
the hormonal influences which result in the menopause
and therefore enable you to explain to your patients what
is happening to their bodies. Later chapters will look in
more depth at the consequences of these changes.

DEFINITIONS

Strictly speaking, the term **menopause** simply means *last menstrual bleed* and as such cannot be diagnosed until after the event.

The phase of time either side of this last bleed is described as the **climacteric** and it is during this time that many women experience physical and psychological symptoms, along with the emotional changes which some women will attribute to 'the menopause'.

In practice, both health professionals and women themselves use the term 'menopause' to include all aspects of this phase of life. Women talk about going 'through the menopause' referring to the months or even years of physical and emotional turmoil which may occur at this time.

A World Health Organization report on the menopause uses the following definitions: (WHO, 1981)

Menopause Permanent cessation of menstruation resulting from the loss of ovarian follicular activity.

Perimenopause (or climacteric) The period immediately prior to menopause with endocrinological, biological and clinical features of approaching menopause and at least the first year after the menopause.

Postmenopause The era following the date of last menstrual bleed which cannot be determined until 12 months of spontaneous amenorrhoea has been observed.

ONSET

In the United Kingdom, the majority of women experience the menopause at around the age of 51 years

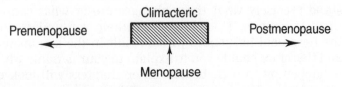

Figure 1.1   Phases of the climacteric.

although it is common for it to occur as early as 45 or as late as 56 years.

Menopause can occur at a very early age in some women, even in the 20s and 30s. This is described as a **premature menopause** and such women deserve special attention, both in terms of physical care and also with regard to emotional support (see Chapter 4).

Age of menopause does not seem to be affected by:

- Race
- Use of oral contraception
- Number of pregnancies
- Age of menarche
- Socioeconomic factors

Smoking however, does appear to bring forward the age of menopause by 1–2 years (Lindquist and Bengrisson, 1979; Sharara et al, 1994).

WHAT HAPPENS AT THE TIME OF THE MENOPAUSE?

Hormonal influences

In order to understand how menopause occurs it is important to have a basic understanding of the normal female physiology, during reproductive years.

During menstruation, low levels of oestrogen and progestogen are released into the bloodstream. The hypothalamus controls the secretions of these hormones through the release of luteinizing hormone releasing hormones (LHRH), which then stimulates the pituitary gland to produce follicle stimulating hormone (FSH). FSH, in turn stimulates the ovaries to produce oestradiol which causes the endometrium to proliferate. As circulating oestradiol increases, FSH and LH levels fall until around day 14 of the cycle. LH then peaks and ovulation generally occurs. If fertilization does not take place, oestrogen and progestogen levels fall and the endometrium is shed – menstruation takes place. The falling levels of oestrogen and progestogen are detected by the hypothalamus and the cycle starts again.

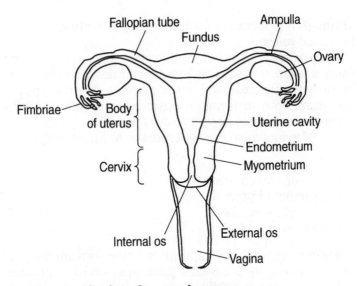

Figure 1.2   The female sexual organs.

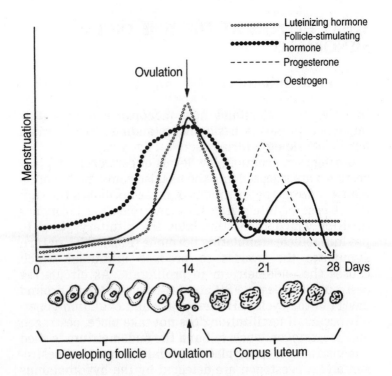

Figure 1.3   Normal menstrual cycle.

From around the age of 35 years, the natural cycle becomes less predictable and ovulation may not occur in every cycle. Oestrogen levels fall and as a result of the negative feedback system of the pituitary and hypothalamus glands, more and more follicle-stimulating hormone is released, in an attempt to stimulate ovarian function. When oestrogen levels fall too low to stimulate endometrial growth, bleeding stops altogether and the menopause occurs.

Follicle stimulating hormone

Hormonal changes begin well before a woman sees an alteration in her menstrual pattern. Fluctuations of follicle stimulating hormone (FSH) and luteinizing hormone (LH) occur throughout the perimenopause, eventually peaking 2–3 years after periods stop and remaining high for the next 20 years or so (unless HRT is taken) (Chakravati et al, 1976).

Oestradiol/oestrone

In the premenopausal woman, both oestradiol and oestrone are present, with oestradiol being the dominant hormone. Both are secreted by the ovaries but oestrone is also available through conversion in fatty tissue of the hormone androstenedione, which is secreted by the adrenal glands. Oestrone is biologically less active than oestradiol. After the menopause, the ratio of oestradiol to oestrone changes with oestrone becoming the dominant hormone.

Measuring Hormones

Many women believe that they need a blood test to confirm whether or not they are menopausal. In practice they are often unnecessary. Symptoms of the menopause do not correlate to actual levels of circulating oestrogen. Some women experience symptoms whilst maintaining relatively high oestrogen levels whilst others, even with lower levels, may not get such bad symptoms.

Table 1.1   Hormone changes following menopause

Hormone	Change in concentration
Oestradiol (E2)	↓
Oestrone (E1)	↓
Ratio of E2:E1	Reverses
FSH	↑
LH	↑

↑, Increase; ↓, decrease

Measurement of FSH will help diagnose menopause but as levels fluctuate widely in the perimenopause, repeated levels would be required to be sure of an accurate result. Measuring FSH or oestradiol will not help in predicting whether or not a woman needs HRT. However FSH levels may be useful in the following circumstances:

- Hysterectomized women (see Chapter 4)
- Diagnosis of premature menopause which may have medical/psychological implications (see Chapter 4)
- To confirm lack of ovarian function for those women seeking advice about contraception (see Chapter 5)

Effect of hysterectomy on menopause

Even if ovaries are conserved at the time of hysterectomy, it is possible that the menopause will occur early (see Chapter 4; Siddle et al, 1987). If a woman experiences an early menopause as a result of her hysterectomy, but is asymptomatic, she could be at increased risk of osteoporosis and cardiovascular disease if that early menopause is not detected.

LIFE EXPECTANCY

Women approaching the menopause can now expect to live for many more years; many women are living into their eighties and beyond. It is therefore becoming

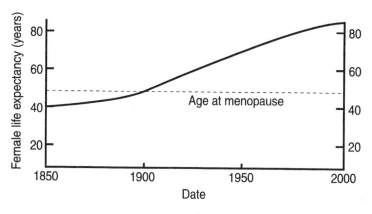

Figure 1.4 Changing life expectancy.

increasingly important to women that the postmenopausal years are as healthy as those before the menopause. Women often ask, 'why must I think about the menopause, when my grandmother just got on with it?' The truth is that far fewer women of her grandmother's generation lived for many years after the menopause. It is not the menopause which has changed in character (although we do have a greater understanding of the physical changes now), but rather that women's expectation of life beyond the menopause has changed.

CONCLUSION

The menopause marks the end of fertility and the end of periods. The menopause itself is merely the outward manifestation of all the hormonal changes which will occur in a women at this time. Helping women to understand the physiological causes of menopause and reminding them how their bodies normally function, is the first step in helping a woman come to terms with her changing body and then with all the other changes which may be occurring at the same time.

REFERENCES

Chakravati S, Collins WP, Newton JR et al (1976) Hormonal profiles after the menopause. *Br. Med. J.* ii: 784.

Lindquist O & Bengrisson C (1979) The effect of smoking on menopausal age. *Maturitas* 1: 191.

Sharara FI, Beatse SN, Leonard MR et al (1994) Cigarettes smoking accelerates the development of diminished ovarian reserve as evidenced by the clomiphene citrate challenge test. *Fertil. Steril.* 62(2): 257–262.

Siddle N, Sarrel P & Whitehead MI (1987) The effect of hysterectomy on the age of ovarian failure: identification of a sub group of women with premature loss of ovarian function. *Fertil. Steril.* 47: 94.

World Health Organization (1981) *Report of a WHO Scientific Group, Research on the Menopause*. WHO Technical Report Series 670, Geneva.

Chapter 2

Short- and Intermediate-term Symptoms

If the menopause simply represented an end to periods and to the possibility of having children, most women would accept it gratefully, even if those feelings were tinged with an element of sadness. An adjustment would be made to a new life era and life would continue.

However, the menopause brings with it agonies as well as blessings! Books and magazines would have women believe that menopausal women are in their 'prime of life', yet distressing symptoms and hormonal upheaval can make a woman feel anything but in her prime. The menopause is often called the 'change of life' and some women would say that it is a change for the worse – distressing symptoms, weak bladders and the beginning of the battle against the ageing process.

Of course, not everything which happens to a woman and her body during mid life can be blamed on the menopause. Hormones play a significant part in physical changes at this time, but some changes are similar in both men and women and cannot be blamed solely on hormones. Other changes may arise as a direct consequence of a less than perfect lifestyle as the effects of smoking or dietary habits may become more obvious. This chapter outlines those symptoms which are commonly identified as being related to the climacteric, both physical and psychological. Long-term consequences of oestrogen deficiency are discussed elsewhere.

INCIDENCE

The list of potential menopausal symptoms appears endless (Fig. 2.1). Fortunately no woman experiences all the symptoms and indeed some women experience no obvious symptoms at all. However it is estimated that 75% of postmenopausal women do experience acute symptoms, often starting before menstruation even stops and sometimes continuing for many years afterwards. Many symptoms are entirely self-limiting with no effect other than mild discomfort to a woman, whilst others become so distressing that they may substantially upset a woman's life.

- 25% of women continue to experience symptoms for 5 years.
- 5% of women are still experiencing symptoms many years after the menopause.
- 51% of symptomatic women describe their symptoms as 'severe'.

(McKinlay and Jeffereys, 1974; Samsioe et al, 1985)

The average length of time that a woman experiences symptoms is around 2 years. Symptoms will come and go in some women, whilst other women will have symptoms more persistently. The severity of symptoms also varies, both among women and even within an individual's own experience (Fig. 2.2). Two women may experience the same degree of symptoms yet one will cope whilst another finds them disruptive to her life. This will

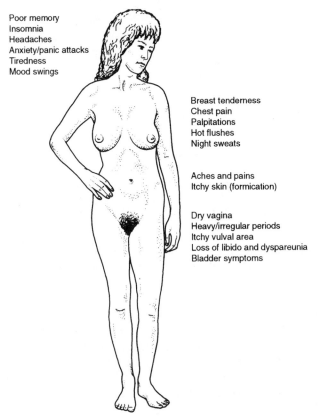

Poor memory
Insomnia
Headaches
Anxiety/panic attacks
Tiredness
Mood swings

Breast tenderness
Chest pain
Palpitations
Hot flushes
Night sweats

Aches and pains
Itchy skin (formication)

Dry vagina
Heavy/irregular periods
Itchy vulval area
Loss of libido and dyspareunia
Bladder symptoms

SHORT TERM
SYMPTOMS
— Incidence
— Vasomotor symptoms

Figure 2.1   Summary of typical symptoms associated with the menopause.

depend on her job and her lifestyle as well as her attitude to the symptoms.

VASOMOTOR SYMPTOMS

The **hot flush** is probably the symptom which is most widely recognized as being menopause-related. Almost all women and many men would be able to associate the hot flush with 'the change'. Hot flushes are extremely common although their frequency and intensity will vary greatly between individuals.

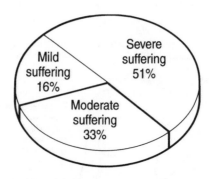

Figure 2.2   Severity of symptoms in menopausal women. (Adapted from Samsioe, 1985, from 'Managing the Menopause II' by Cathy Read.)

Women describe a hot flush as a feeling of intense heat, sometimes accompanied by sweating, starting in the chest area and rising through the neck and face. When flushes occur at night, they often manifest as **night sweats,** causing a woman to wake feeling most uncomfortable and very hot and sweaty. These can continue for many months, night after night, leaving the woman feeling both physically tired and emotionally drained as a result of lack of sleep. This can cause stress in a relationship between partners, particularly if it continues for a long time.

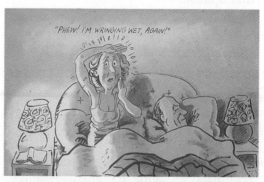

Figure 2.3   Night sweats can lead a woman to feel physically and emotionally drained. (From slide set 'Understanding the Menopause' by permission of Wyeth Laboratories.)

The actual cause of hot flushes is unclear. They are not related to specific levels of oestrogen in the blood, but rather to the rate of change. This would explain why they are most common in the early stages of the climacteric – the time of greatest hormonal upheaval.

Flushes and sweats are not life-threatening but they can be very distressing. Many women are affected at work, causing embarrassment and difficulty. Home and leisure activities are also affected. Fortunately, flushes respond well to hormone replacement therapy (Coope et al, 1975). Within 2–3 weeks of starting treatment, flushes and sweats should be improved and if an adequate dose of oestrogen is given they should disappear altogether. Nonhormonal methods of relieving flushes and sweats are discussed in Chapter 8. Hot flushes can be worsened by:

- Hot and spicy foods
- Alcohol intake
- Cigarette smoking
- Caffeine intake
- Hot weather

Hot flushes may be associated with **palpitations**, which can lead to symptoms of anxiety as women worry that there is something seriously wrong with their heart.

MUSCLE AND JOINT PAINS

Many women complain of generalized aches and pains around the time of the climacteric. It is often impossible to say whether such symptoms are in fact hormonally related. Hormone replacement therapy (HRT) is sometimes beneficial, perhaps by improving the collagen content of ligaments and connective tissue. HRT will not reverse the effects of osteoarthritis which is a common complaint in older women.

SKIN SYMPTOMS

Women on HRT often describe a change in their skin elasticity which is probably due to a beneficial effect on the collagen content. Changes in the skin at the time of the menopause can lead to:

- Loss of elasticity/suppleness
- Dry skin
- Formication (intense tingling or sensation of crawling on the skin)

BLADDER SYMPTOMS

Bladder symptoms are commonly experienced by perimenopausal women. However it is difficult to differentiate between those symptoms which are genuinely hormone-related and those which are caused by general ageing factors. It is true that women are often more aware of their symptoms at around the time of the menopause, with one study showing that 50% of women attending a menopause clinic had urinary symptoms (Cardozo, 1990). However whether the menopause itself has actually caused the problems is unclear. Oestrogen and progestogen receptors have been found in the urethra and the bladder, so it is likely that they will be sensitive to hormone changes (Versi and Cardozo, 1988). Typical bladder symptoms are:

- Stress incontinence
- Frequency of micturition
- Urgency of micturition
- Nocturia

Women are often embarrassed to talk about bladder problems, so sympathetic questioning may be required. A trial of oestrogen therapy may be beneficial. Nocturia, urgency and urge incontinence may be helped by oestrogen, whereas the condition of genuine stress incontinence is not thought to be helped by oestrogen (Versi, 1994). Referral for urodynamic studies should be considered in those women in whom bladder symptoms are severe enough to affect their normal daily activities (J. Pitkin, pers. commun.). Women should not feel that such symptoms must simply be tolerated as an inevitable part of middle age.

SEXUAL FUNCTION

A common misconception is that the menopause marks the end of sexual fulfilment for women. Many women expect problems to begin at this time and therefore have a lower expectation of sexual enjoyment. It is true that in the years immediately preceding and following the menopause, some women experience changes in their sexual function. Such changes may include:

- Decreased sexual desire
- Diminished sexual response
- Loss of libido

(Sarrel, 1988)

However some women will find that their sex life improves rather than declines after the menopause. Both hormonal and nonhormonal factors will influence sexual function at the time of the menopause.

Oestrogen lack

Declining oestrogen levels at the time of the menopause and thereafter (unless HRT is taken), result in profound changes to the vagina and vulval areas. Atrophic changes result in a shorter, less elastic vagina with less vascularity and a thinner and more easily irritated epithelium – **atrophic vaginitis**. This can lead to **vaginal dryness** and **dyspareunia** (painful intercourse). This inevitably stops a women from enjoying lovemaking to the full and can result in both physical and psychological problems. Vaginal secretions diminish and the vagina becomes more susceptible to infection because of a changing pH. Changes in the vagina due to oestrogen deficiency are:

- Increased pH – less resistance to infection
- Decreased blood flow
- Loss of elasticity
- Shortens in length
- Loss of muscle tone
- Decreased cervical secretion

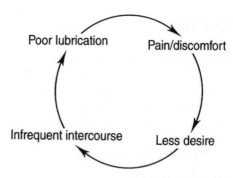

Figure 2.4   Cycle demonstrating sexual difficulties.

Replacing oestrogen either systemically or locally will help to maintain vaginal lubrication and then to assist in making sexual intercourse more comfortable.

Anxiety

If sexual intercourse is painful or results in bleeding, a woman may become anxious and tense, which will make her next attempt at intercourse less successful. A cycle can be established such as shown in Fig. 2.4.

Body image

The climacteric can be a time when a woman has to confront the fact that she is ageing. The cessation of menstruation is tangible evidence that the reproductive phase is over. For some women this is a relief; contraception is no longer required and sex can be enjoyed simply for its own sake. Women with this attitude may expect to continue a satisfying sex life well into their postmenopausal years and indeed, continuing sexual intercourse after the menopause may in itself help to prevent atrophic changes (Leiblum et al, 1983).

Other women consider the menopause to be a step toward old age, a time of deterioration in health, both physical and sexual. Such an attitude can cause a psychological barrier to continuing sexual relations. Negative self image can contribute to a sense of feeling nonsexual and therefore to a loss of desire for sexual activity (Sarrel and Whitehead, 1985). This is discussed further in Chapter 5.

The male partner

Problems with sexual activity around mid life are not necessarily a simple result of hormonal changes in the woman. The male partner may also be developing problems such as erectile difficulty or loss of desire. These may be contributing to a less than satisfying sexual relationship. Satisfaction within the relationship, emotional stability and psychological well-being will all contribute to a healthy and satisfying sex life. If a problem exists it will probably exist for both partners although they may be affected in different ways. Both partners therefore need to be involved in any discussion or treatment suggestions.

Psychosexual counselling

Some couples will need specific counselling and help in their relationship. Such counselling will involve:

- Careful and attentive listening
- Provision of information about sexual function
- Reassurance
- Suggestions for improving communication about one's feelings
- Encouragement to re-establish sexual activity when appropriate

(Sarrel, 1988)

For most women, a combination of counselling, reassurance and HRT if appropriate, will be sufficient for a couple to resolve sexual difficulties. A few women may need referral to a sex therapist for more in-depth treatment.

PSYCHOLOGICAL SYMPTOMS

In addition to physical symptoms, some women experience emotional or psychological symptoms around the time of the menopause. Many women do not understand that such feelings may occur and become very anxious about them. Typical psychological symptoms are:

- Panic attacks
- Poor memory
- Lack of concentration
- Irritability
- Mood swings
- Anxiety
- Depressed mood
- Fatigue

Despite many studies, it has proved difficult to ascertain whether these symptoms are truly endocrine effects or whether they arise as a result of compounding factors affecting a woman at this time. Mid life is often a time of social and emotional upheaval and the following may be contributory factors to psychological symptoms:

- Marriage difficulties
- Divorce
- Children leaving home
- Change in work/home responsibilities
- Death or illness in the family

These factors are discussed more fully in Chapter 5.

Nevertheless some studies have shown that minor psychological complaints can correlate to fluctuating oestrogen levels (Ballinger, 1975; Montgomery et al, 1987). Hunter et al (1986) showed that in a study of 850 women, depressed mood, and sleep problems were more common in the perimenopausal era than premenopausally. This confirmed the work of earlier studies (Thompson et al, 1973; Ballinger, 1975).

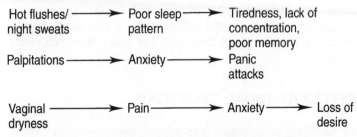

Figure 2.5   Examples of the domino effect.

Table 2.1 Summary of typical effects of oestrogen deficiency

Short term	Flushes/sweats
	Psychological complaints
	Insomnia
	Joint pains
Intermediate	Vaginal symptoms
	Bladder symptoms
	Sexual difficulties
Long term	Osteoporosis
	Cardiovascular disease

The 'Domino effect' has also been described (Whitehead and Godfree, 1992). Psychological effects may arise from the physical symptoms of the climacteric (Fig. 2.5).

It is unlikely that all psychological symptoms attributed to 'the change' are truly hormone-related, but rather that there is an interaction between physical and psychological factors affecting women at this time. Women may be more prone to psychological symptoms during the climacteric if they have a past history of psychiatric disease or if they experience difficulty in coping with stress (Hunter, 1988).

Effect of HRT on psychological symptoms

HRT may help psychological symptoms as well as physical ones. Campbell and Whitehead (1977) found that oestrogen was significantly more effective than placebo in alleviating symptoms such as anxiety, poor memory, irritability and insomnia. Some of the women in this study did not experience hot flushes so the assumption is that the beneficial effect was direct rather than through the domino effect. Women with severe physical symptoms, relieved by HRT, often describe psychological improvement as well, highlighting the obvious interaction between the physical and the psychological.

Psychological symptoms can cause a woman great anxiety so reassurance and explanations are an impor-

SHORT TERM SYMPTOMS – Psychological symptoms

tant part of her care. Nonhormonal therapies for relief of psychological symptoms are discussed in Chapter 8.

The effects of menopausal symptoms are often underestimated by health professionals. Women often say that they do not feel that they are taken seriously by their doctor or that they (the patient) do not want to 'trouble' the doctor over something which is distressing but not life-threatening. However, for some women, these symptoms will affect not just their home life, but their work and their relationships too. It is therefore important that women are encouraged at least to discuss their symptoms, even if they ultimately decide to persevere with them and not take HRT. Reassurance that typical symptoms are normal is sometimes enough. Lack of information and knowledge will lead only to further anxiety. Women need more information both about typical menopausal symptoms and about treatment which may be available for them.

REFERENCES

Ballinger CB (1975) Psychiatric morbidity and the menopause screening of general population: sample. *Br. Med J.* 3: 344.

Campbell S & Whitehead MI (1977) Oestrogen therapy and the menopausal syndrome. *Clin. Obstet. Gynaecol.* 4: 31–47.

Cardozo L (1990) Oestrogen deficiency and the bladder. In Drife JO & Studd JWW (eds) *HRT and Osteoporosis*. London: Springer-Verlag.

Coope J, Thompson JM & Poller L (1975) Effect of 'natural oestrogen' replacement therapy on menopausal symptoms and blood clotting. *Br. Med. J.* 4: 139.

Hunter M (1988) Psychological aspects of the climacteric. In Studd JWW & Whitehead MI (eds) *The Menopause*. Oxford: Blackwell Scientific.

Hunter M, Battersby R & Whitehead MI (1986) Relationships between psychological symptoms, somatic complaints and menopause status. *Maturitas* 8: 217–218.

Leiblum SR, Bachmann GA, Kemmann E et al (1983) Vaginal atrophy in the post menopausal woman. *J. Am. Med. Assoc.* 249: 2195–2198.

McKinlay SM & Jeffreys M (1974) The menopausal syndrome. *Br. J. Prevent. Med.* 28: 108.

Montgomery JC, Appleby L, Brincat M et al (1987) Effects of oestrogen and testosterone implant therapy on psychological disorders in the climacteric. *Lancet* i: 297.

Samsioe G, Bryman I & Ivansson E (1985) Some anthropological aspects of the climacteric syndrome. *Acta Obstet. Gynaecol. Scand.*, **130** (suppl.): 5.

Sarrel PM (1988) Sexuality. In Studd JWW & Whitehead MI (eds) *The Menopause.* Oxford: Blackwell Scientific.

Sarrel PM & Whitehead MI (1985) Sex and the menopause: defining the issues. *Maturitas* **7**: 217–224.

Thompson B, Hart SA & Durno D (1973) Menopausal age and symptomatology in general practice. *J. Biol. Soc. Sci.* **5**: 71–82.

Versi E (1994) Ageing and hormonal changes of the bladder and urethra. *Curr. Prob. Obstet. Gynaecol. Fertil.* **17**: 193–232.

Versi E & Cardozo LD (1988) Oestrogens and the lower urinary tract function. In Studd JWW & Whitehead MI (eds) *The Menopause.* Oxford: Blackwell Scientific.

Whitehead MI & Godfree V (1992) HRT – your questions answered. London: Churchill Livingstone.

Chapter 3

Long-term Consequences of Oestrogen Deficiency

It is probably true to say that women are most concerned about the immediate effects of the menopause on their lives – the symptoms, be they physical or psychological. When symptoms become disruptive to their lives, they will seek help. HRT looks more attractive to a woman when she can see the tangible benefits she may enjoy. Yet, from a medical perspective, these symptoms are usually harmless. They can cause a lot of discomfort, embarrassment and heartache, but are seldom life-threatening in themselves. Many will disappear spontaneously if left untreated, although it may take several years. For many women, months or even years of their lives will be spoiled so it is very important that even short-term HRT is made available to them if appropriate.

In the long term, however, women's bodies do change as a result of oestrogen deficiency. The skeleton and the cardiovascular system are the most readily identified as changing after the menopause, but it is possible that many other body systems are affected. One area which is being researched at present is that of the brain, in relation to **Alzheimer's disease**. There is evidence that oestrogen may affect the part of the brain responsible for cholinergic neurotransmitters, which regulate cognitive functions. Early studies are encouraging, but larger scale, prospective studies are required (Paginini-Hill and Henderson, 1994; Barrett-Connor and Kritz-Silverstein, 1993).

The evidence for the effects on the skeletal and cardiovascular systems are more widely accepted and so this chapter concentrates on these.

OSTEOPOROSIS

Osteoporosis is not a new problem. However as life expectancy improves and with more and more elderly people living in our society, awareness of this disease is becoming important. Although prevalence of osteoporosis among men is increasing too, it is principally the female population who need a greater understanding of the disease and how they might be affected. Oestrogen deficiency is the main cause of osteoporosis in women, arising as a consequence of the menopause, although it is often not until many years later that the effects are seen. It is the more elderly women who commonly experience fractures relating to osteoporosis (Grimley-Evans et al, 1979). Yet if the disease is to be prevented, then measures need to be taken at a much earlier stage in life. Whilst it is never too late to try to minimize the effects of osteoporosis, it is wise to start early and in particular to consider the time of the menopause as an important stage in the development of the disease. This section will look at what osteoporosis is, how it may be prevented and how HRT may be of benefit. It will also cover briefly other treatments for osteoporosis and suggest some ways of managing the effects of the disease once it is established.

Definition

Osteoporosis is a condition in which the structure of the bone (or 'bone mass') weakens to such an extent that the risk of fracture is greatly increased. These fractures occur not as a result of major trauma, but following trivial accidents or even during everyday activities. For example, an elderly woman might simply step off the kerb and fracture a hip, or bend down in the garden and suffer a spinal fracture. Women who are at risk of such fractures would be said to have osteoporosis even if they have not yet experienced a fracture. If they have already experienced a fracture they may be described as having 'established osteoporosis'.

The ageing process

Throughout life, bone is continually renewed and replaced. During childhood and young adulthood there is a net increase in bone density, resulting in skeletal growth. At around the age of 35 years, peak bone mass is achieved and less bone formation takes place. This results in an overall decline in bone density as we get older (Fig. 3.1). This process occurs in both men and women and is related to age (Riggs et al, 1982). Women

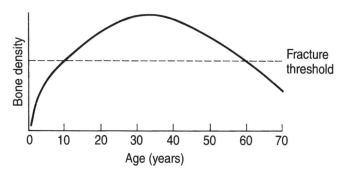

Figure 3.1   Change of bone density with age.

also demonstrate an additional rapid decline in bone density around the time of the menopause and for several years afterwards (Stevenson et al, 1989). It is this sudden decrease in bone density which can cause a woman to fall below the so-called **fracture threshold** later in life.

One aim of any osteoporosis prevention strategy is to prevent bone density falling below this fracture threshold, thus ideally preventing fractures occurring. Long-term strategies also include trying to improve peak bone mass in young adults. This means that the prevention of osteoporosis should be taken seriously throughout life.

Normal bone structure

Bone is a living part of the body, being constantly removed and renewed. Cells in bone structure are responsible for this turnover, with the two main cells being **osteoblasts** and **osteoclasts**. Osteoblasts replace and renew bone, whilst osteoclasts remove old bone. If both are in balance bone density is maintained. If osteoclasts remove bone faster than osteoblasts can replace it then bone density is reduced, leaving the overall structure of the bone weakened. Bone is not a solid structure, but is made up of a network of fibres, criss-crossing each other to maintain strength. Osteoporotic bone has less strength because the criss-cross structures become broken or decayed, causing the overall structure to be weakened (Fig. 3.2).

The strength of the skeleton at a given time will depend on the **bone density**, or **bone mass**. This will be at its peak at around the mid-thirties, declining gradually thereafter. Peak bone mass (i.e. the maximum to be achieved) is influenced by the following factors:

- Race
- Genetic factors
- Hormonal influences
- Diet
- Smoking

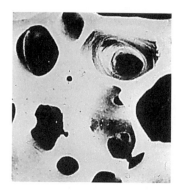 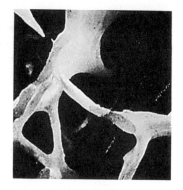

Figure 3.2   Electron micrograph showing normal and osteoporotic bone. Reproduced from Dempster et al (1986) with permission. © Elsevier Science Inc.

Incidence

Osteoporotic fractures are extremely common. Each year there are approximately 200 000 fractures of the hip, wrist and spine, the majority of which are likely to have been caused by osteoporosis. The three commonest sites for fracture as a result of osteoporosis are the wrist, spine and hip (Fig. 3.3).

Wrist

Each year there are about 40 000 cases of fracture of the distal forearm, often resulting from a fall on to an outstretched hand. The rate of these fractures rises in woman after the age of 50 until around the age of 65 years. There is no corresponding increase seen in men at this age. After the age of 65 years there appears to be no further rise in the rate of these fractures among women (Stevenson and Marsh, 1992).

Hip

The incidence of hip fracture among elderly women is remarkably high and they are potentially very serious. Approximately one third of women who sustain a hip

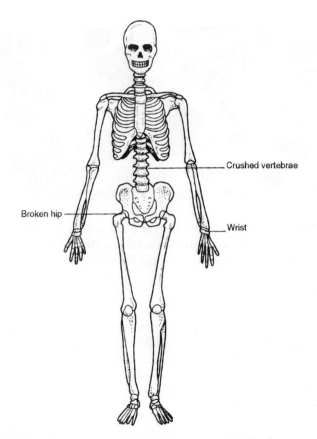

Broken hip

Crushed vertebrae

Wrist

Figure 3.3   Common sites for osteoporotic fracture.

fracture will die within 1 year (Grimley-Evans et al, 1979) and about a half go on to suffer long-term pain and disability. Treatment of hip fractures is by surgical fixation which carries the immediate risk associated with general anaesthesia and the longer-term risks associated with immobility in an already elderly or frail person.

Incidence of hip fractures is likely to increase as a result of a rise in the number of elderly people in our population (Grimley-Evans, 1990).

Spine

Vertebral fractures occur when osteoporosis causes the vertebral bodies to collapse, causing a 'wedging'. Inci-

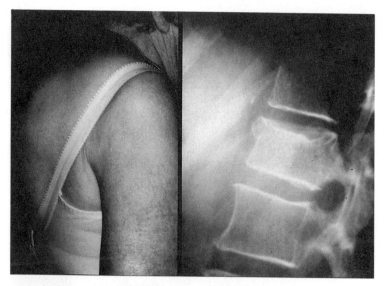

Figure 3.4   Woman with severe osteoporosis. Reproduced from 'Talking to patients about the menopause and HRT', with permission of Medipic/P. Stott.

dence of these fractures is difficult to assess because they often occur silently and are only demonstrated on X-ray at a much later stage. It has been estimated that only one third of such fractures are brought to medical attention at the actual time of fracture (Grimley-Evans, 1990). Sudden acute fractures of the vertebra cause intense pain, requiring urgent medical help. The so called 'Dowagers hump' or **kyphosis**, arises after repeated vertebral fractures (Fig. 3.5).

Causes

Osteoporosis can be caused by various factors. Peak bone mass is achieved by early adulthood and is largely genetically predetermined. Lifestyle factors such as diet and exercise may also influence the development of the skeleton (Kandlers et al, 1984; Kanis and Passmore, 1989). Race is also an influencing factor: black women have a greater bone density than whites and Asians (Cohn et al, 1977).

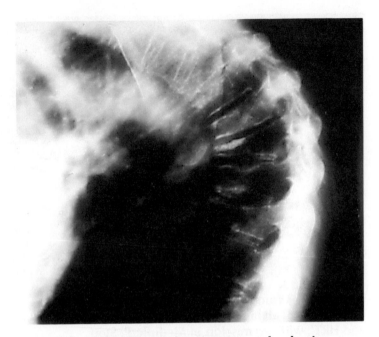

**Figure 3.5   Spinal X-ray showing severe kyphosis.
(Reproduced with permission of Wyeth Laboratories.)**

Whether or not a woman suffers osteoporosis will
depend not only on how good a peak bone mass she
achieves as a young adult but also on the rate at which
she loses bone density later in life. The initial 5–10 years
following the menopause is a time of rapid bone loss in
women, but the actual rate of loss will vary from woman
to woman (Johnstone et al, 1985). A woman might
achieve an excellent peak bone mass, but subsequently
lose bone very quickly, putting her at as much risk as a
woman who achieves a low peak bone mass but who then
loses at a much slower rate.

Whilst osteoporosis is commonly a result of oestrogen
deficiency at the time of the menopause, it can also occur
as a result of the following factors:

- Corticosteroid therapy (above 75 mg prednisolone
  daily or equivalent dose, on a regular basis)
- Hyperparathyroidism

- Cushing's syndrome
- Some malignant diseases
- Long-term immobilization
- Excessive exercise, as in athletes or ballet dancers
- Chronic hepatic or renal failure
- Rheumatoid arthritis

Risk factors

Various risk factors have been identified which are thought to predict those women who may be at an increased risk of developing osteoporosis and therefore who might experience fractures later in life. Identifying those women at risk would mean that intervention strategies could be targetted and those women most likely to be at risk of fracture in the future could receive treatment. Known risk factors are:

- Race
- Family history
- Early menopause
- High alcohol intake
- Cigarette smoking
- Low body weight
- Episodes of amenorrhoea
- Nulliparity
- Long-term corticosteroid therapy
- Sedentary lifestyle

Studies have shown, however, that risk factors such as these are not good predictors of future risk of fracture (Wasnich et al, 1987). It has been estimated that by using these risk factors, only about 30% of people will be identified, who will subsequently develop osteoporosis (Stevenson et al, 1989). In the absence of other more accurate methods of predicting risk, these factors can sometimes be the only indication of whether a woman is potentially at risk. It is considered far more accurate to actually measure the bone density in order to predict future risk of fracture.

Measuring bone density

When trying to assess an individual woman and predict her risk of fracture, it is helpful to be able to measure bone density. Risk of fracture has been demonstrated to be greatest in women who have the lowest bone density (Leichter et al, 1982). Measuring bone density also enables doctors to be selective in their treatments and only treat those women who would appear to be in need of intervention therapy. This is in contrast to the common situation where women are often offered HRT as a 'precaution' against osteoporosis even though they have not actually been demonstrated to be at high risk of fracture. Women themselves would probably feel more confident in the need for treatment and compliance rates for therapy would probably improve. Measurement of bone density can be performed by the following methods:

- Conventional X-ray
- Single photon absorbtiometry
- Dual photon absorbtiometry
- Dual energy X-ray absorbtiometry
- Quantitative computed tomography
- Ultrasound

X-ray

Conventional radiography only shows a profound loss of bone density. It is therefore of little value in assessing a woman's risk of osteoporosis. By the time the loss of bone density is demonstrated by X-ray, the disease is well established and treatment more difficult. It is more usual for X-ray to be used simply as a tool for diagnosis of fractures, rather than as an assessment of risk of osteoporosis.

Single photon absorbtiometry (SPA)

SPA was the earliest way of measuring bone density. Measurement is of the forearm, which whilst useful, does not always give an indication of osteoporosis at other sites. Measurement of the hip and spine is not possible with SPA.

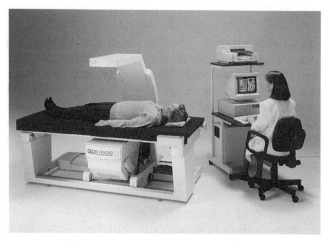

Figure 3.6   DEXA machine. (Reproduced with permission of Vertec Scientific.)

Dual photon absorbtiometry (DPA)

DPA measures bone density in both the femur and lumbar spine, as well as in the total body. It gives a more accurate reading than SPA. Scanning time with DPA is about 20 minutes each for hip and spine.

Dual energy X-ray absorbtiometry (DEXA)

This is similar to DPA but with greater precision. Scanning time is only about 15 minutes at each site and radiation doses are smaller (Stevenson and Marsh, 1992). DEXA (Fig. 3.6) has generally replaced the use of DPA as a diagnostic tool. Newer machines will make scanning time even shorter.

Quantitative computed tomography (QCT)

QCT is used to measure bone density in the spine. It uses larger doses of radiation and is considerably more expensive than other methods. It is often used for research purposes.

Ultrasound

Ultrasound technique can be used to measure bone density in the heel. A low bone density in the heel appears to correlate to a low bone density in the hip or spine (Argen et al, 1991). Potentially this simple method of measurement could be widely used as a tool for assessing risk of osteoporosis or for identifying those women who require further investigation.

Why measure bone density?

Measurement of bone density at around the time of the menopause will help to identify whether a woman is at risk of fracture later in life (Hui et al, 1988). A further scan 12–18 months later will also help assess the actual rate of bone loss over this period of time. Such measurements are particularly useful for the woman who is re luctant to take HRT but who is concerned abou osteoporosis. If a bone density measurement clearly shows an increased risk, it is much easier for the woman to understand the need for her HRT and will help her to make an informed decision. Repeat scans can also encourage a woman to remain on therapy because there is tangible evidence of the benefits. In high risk women it can ensure that the doses of treatment given are sufficient for protection in that individual woman.

So far there is insufficient evidence to support widespread screening of all women, as a cost-effective and efficient exercise. However research is underway to look at this issue. Meanwhile on an individual basis, bone density measurements can be helpful, particularly in highlighting those women who would not consider HRT except for prevention of osteoporosis.

On the NHS?

To date bone density measurements are not always available on the NHS. Many health authorities do have the necessary equipment and staff to provide this service, but in some parts of the country the test may only be available privately or as part of a research programme.

The Department of Health supports the use of bone density as a means to assess patients on an individual basis and has recommended that facilities should be available (DOH, 1994).

In order to clarify who is eligible for bone density measurement on the NHS, some health authorities have drawn up clear guidelines so that there is no confusion amongst local doctors. These guidelines are often based on the known risk factors for the disease, so whilst most women at risk should be eligible, there will inevitably be some women who do not appear to be at risk and are therefore not measured.

The role of calcium

Many women believe that if they simply take extra calcium at the time of the menopause, they will prevent osteoporosis. Calcium, like all vitamins and minerals, is an essential part of a healthy diet. The majority of women who eat a well balanced diet will not benefit simply by taking calcium supplements. It certainly cannot halt the rapid loss of bone density which occurs at the time of the menopause (Heaney, 1987). One study has shown that elderly women who have a poor calcium intake may benefit from calcium supplements and see a slight rise in density (Dawson-Hughes et al, 1991).

A healthy diet should be encouraged and women who eat very few dairy products may be deficient in calcium if they are not taking it in other foods. These women should be advised about the possible need for dietary supplements (see Chapter 8).

Exercise

Regular weight-bearing exercise, such as walking or jogging, produces a small increase in bone density in postmenopausal women (Chow et al, 1987; Stevenson et al, 1989). However it cannot prevent the rapid bone loss experienced at the time of the menopause. Exercise improves flexibility, muscle tone and general fitness, perhaps reducing the likelihood of a fall.

LONG-TERM CONSEQUENCES — Osteoporosis

Table 3.1   Minimum doses of oestrogen required for bone preservation

Oestrogen	Dose (mg)
Conjugated oestrogens	0.625 mg
Oral oestradiol	2 mg
Transdermal oestradiol	50 μg
Oestradiol valerate	2 mg

Exercise is always to be commended but should be used in conjunction with other therapies rather than in place of them (Stevenson and Marsh, 1992).

Excessive exercise such as that undertaken by athletes or ballet dancers in training is harmful to bone, resulting in a low premenopausal bone density, which will increase the risk of fracture in later life, particularly following a further rapid loss at the time of the menopause (Drinkwater et al, 1984). This is likely to be due to low oestrogen levels which often occur in these women, leading to prolonged episodes of amenorrhoea or oligomenorrhoea.

HRT AND OSTEOPOROSIS

Retrospective studies have shown that 5 years use of oestrogen therapy is associated with a halving in the risk of hip fracture (Paginini-Hill et al, 1981). Vertebral fracture risk is also reduced (Ettinger et al, 1985). These results indicate that when considering the use of HRT as a protection against osteoporosis, long-term treatment is recommended. Women should be aware that taking HRT for only a few months is unlikely to confer much benefit. Oestrogens may reduce the rate of fracture by increasing mobility and dexterity as well as known direct effects of oestrogen on bone cells.

Studies have demonstrated that implants, patches and tablets all have the effect of preserving bone density, although the required dose of each will vary (Table 3.1) (Stevenson et al, 1990). A small number of women may need higher doses of oestrogen in order to prevent bone loss, but without bone density measurement it is difficult to know who they are.

When to start HRT

For the greatest benefit to the skeleton, HRT should be started soon after the menopause and continue for 5 years (Ettinger et al, 1985). This is the phase of rapid bone loss and it is valuable to conserve bone at this stage, before too much bone density is lost. If HRT is started many years after the menopause, bone density will still be preserved but at a lower level because the woman will have already experienced some bone loss. Some would argue that starting HRT at this point may be sufficient to prevent a fracture occurring so should still be considered valuable. However, fear of potential side-effects and worries about bleeding often put older women off the idea of using HRT.

What happens when HRT is stopped?

When HRT is stopped, bone density declines, but usually at the same rate as immediately after the menopause. The rapid loss experienced at this time is thus delayed by the length of time a woman took HRT (Lindsay et al, 1978; Christiansen et al, 1981). Once a woman stops HRT she loses the protective effect and bone density will decrease, rapidly initially then more slowly. It is not currently clear how long a woman would need to stay on HRT in order to see sustained benefit into her seventies and beyond.

OTHER TREATMENTS FOR OSTEOPOROSIS

Not all women want to take HRT and indeed some women are unable to because of medical contraindications. For these women, lifestyle changes are certainly a step in the right direction, particularly when considering preventing the disease. Those women who are shown already to have osteoporosis may be offered alternative treatments:

- Calcitonin
- Fluoride
- Anabolic steroids

- Bisphosphonates
- Vitamin D

Calcitonin

Calcitonin has been shown to maintain bone density and in some studies actually to increase it (Gruber et al, 1984). It works similarly to oestrogen, by inhibiting osteoclast activity. Its main drawback (apart from cost) is that in the UK it is currently administered by intramuscular injection. Research is underway to look at calcitonin delivered by nasal spray. This form of treatment may offer an alternative to the woman at a high risk of osteoporosis but who cannot take HRT.

Fluoride

Fluoride stimulates bone formation, particularly in the spine, although the response rate between patients varies considerably (Baud et al, 1988). The usual dose is 20–60 mg daily, given with calcium supplementation. It has a number of side-effects, such as gastric upset and limb pains, so careful monitoring is essential. Fluoride is not commonly prescribed, except under close supervision of a specialist. There is concern that bone formed following fluoride therapy may be more susceptible to fracture because of increased fragility. Further studies are required.

Anabolic steroids

Anabolic steroids are occasionally used in patients with osteoporosis. In younger patients it is usual to prescribe it for only a short time, because of potential adverse lipid changes. Side-effects include hirsutism, fluid retention and a deepening of the voice (Stevenson and Marsh, 1992).

Bisphosphonates

These are a group of drugs which are thought to work on bone in a similar way to HRT, yet are nonhormonal. **Disodium etidronate** was the first bisphosphonate to become available for treatment of established spinal osteoporosis. It is a cyclical therapy, with etidronate 400 mg daily orally for 14 days, followed by calcium citrate, 500 mg a day for a further 76 days, making a 90-day cycle, which is then repeated for 3–5 years. Side-effects are rare, with nausea and diarrhoea being occasionally reported. It is recommended that etidronate be taken in the middle of a 4-hour fast, i.e. 2 hours before and 2 hours after food. This is to aid absorption. Another bisphosphonate, alendrolate is also available, which is taken on a continuous basis. Other bisphosphonates are being researched.

Vitamin D

Women who are housebound or institutionalized and who rarely get outside into natural daylight may suffer vitamin D deficiency. This can be corrected by giving supplements at a dose of 400–800 i.u. daily. However research is contradictory as to whether vitamin D is of value in either the prevention or treatment of osteoporosis.

Whilst alternative treatments are continually being researched, HRT remains the treatment option for most postmenopausal women at risk or suffering from osteoporosis.

PAIN RELIEF

The early stages of osteoporosis are not painful. Once fracture has occurred it can be very painful indeed. Hip fractures are treated surgically, but spinal fractures cannot be operated on and for a few weeks after the fracture, immense pain can be present. In some women pain persists and becomes difficult to manage. Whilst considering all the treatment options, it is important to take a serious assessment of pain and suggest ways of relieving it. As well as conventional analgesia the following could be considered:

- Physiotherapy
- Transelectrical nerve stimulation (TENS)
- Acupuncture
- Relaxation

- 'Alternative' therapies
- Advice on coping with daily activities

NATIONAL OSTEOPOROSIS SOCIETY

The National Osteoporosis Society, set up in 1986, is a national charity working for osteoporosis sufferers. As well as providing general information and advice, it has produced a variety of booklets on subjects relating to osteoporosis. These include:

- General information about osteoporosis
- How to cope
- Calcium guide
- Fashion advice for sufferers
- Treatments
- Exercise and physiotherapy
- Pain relief
- HRT

The National Osteoporosis Society is an excellent source of accurate information for both patients and professionals. There is a scientific membership for medical professionals, providing details of conferences and study days as well as providing an update on research into osteoporosis. See the Appendix for the address.

CARDIOVASCULAR DISEASE

In the past most health education programmes relating to heart disease have been aimed at men. The stereotype 'executive flyer' who smokes, drinks, eats too many corporate lunches and who never exercises has been targetted, with the aim of reducing the overall number of deaths from heart disease. At the age of 45 years, men are up to six times more likely than women to die from a heart attack, yet after this age rates among women rise rapidly and by the late sixties, death rates in men and women are equal (Fig. 3.7). Heart disease is the major cause of death in women over the age of 50 years in the UK (DOH, 1994). This increase is considered to be partly

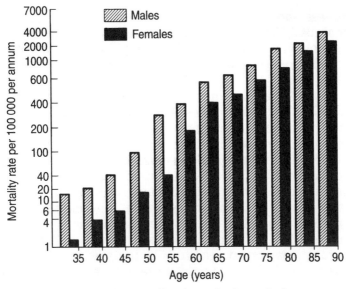

Figure 3.7   Annual mortality from ischaemic heart disease, England and Wales, 1982.

due to falling oestrogen levels and the role they play in relation to heart disease in women.

Significance of the menopause

Whilst it is recognized that ageing alone is a risk factor for cardiovascular disease, it is clear that hormonal status plays an important role in the incidence of cardio-vascular disease in women. In early US studies, it was demonstrated that among groups of women in the same age band, the ones who were postmenopausal had a higher rate of cardiovascular disease than those who still had functioning ovaries (Gordon et al, 1978). This was even more marked among the younger postmenopausal women (Rosenberg et al, 1981).

HRT AND CARDIOVASCULAR DISEASE

Studies have shown that the use of oestrogen therapy after the menopause reduces the risk of both heart disease and stroke (Stamfer and Colditz, 1991; Finucane et al, 1993). There is also evidence to show that menopausal women with established coronary heart disease may benefit from the use of oestrogen therapy (Sullivan et al, 1990).

To date there has not been a large, randomized, controlled study to prove these benefits, but the epidemiological evidence is convincing with many large studies showing a consistent finding, that oestrogen users have a lower risk of developing heart disease than those women not using HRT. Critics would argue that HRT users are not 'typical' women – they may have a high level of contact with medical professionals, they may have an improved general health and they may already have been 'pre-selected' as being fit for oestrogen use. All these factors, it is argued, lead to HRT users being at a lower risk of heart disease than non-users. Three of the largest studies, The Nurses Health Study (Stampfer et al, 1985), The Leisure World Study (Henderson et al, 1991), and the Lipid Research Clinic Follow-up Study (Bush et al, 1987) all showed that cardiovascular risk factors were similar in both users of oestrogen and non-users. These studies show that HRT appears to be a significant protective factor against heart disease in postmenopausal women.

Progestogens

The women in the large scale studies which showed a protective benefit of HRT on the cardiovascular system, have used oestrogen only therapy. With progestogens now routinely added to treatment regimens in the UK, the big question is whether the use of progestogen negates the cardiovascular benefits. Progestogens may have a less favourable effect on blood lipids but this will vary according to the type and dose of progestogen (Lobo, 1991). Few studies are available demonstrating the use of oestrogen/progestogen regimens but a study in 1992 in Sweden showed a 50% reduction in the risk of myocardial infarction in users of a combined therapy (Falkeborn et al, 1992). This indicates that the overall benefits of oestrogen are not necessarily lost with the addition of progestogen. Further studies are needed.

Why is oestrogen beneficial?

Although the scientific evidence shows that oestrogen reduces the risk of cardiovascular disease, it is still unclear as to the precise way in which it works. The following ways have been suggested:

- Beneficial changes in lipid subfractions
- Effects on clotting factors
- Direct effects on blood vessel walls
- Positive changes in insulin metabolism
- Redistribution of body fat

Lipids

After the menopause, changes occur in relation to lipids and lipoproteins which are thought to influence the onset of cardiovascular disease (Table 3.2; Stevenson et al, 1993).

Oestrogen therapy reduces total cholesterol and concentrations of LDL, whilst increasing HDL. This benefit is seen within weeks of starting therapy but does not appear to persist after therapy has been stopped (Stampfer, 1994). Transdermal therapy will not alter HDL although there is a change on subfractions of HDL. Higher concentrations of HDL are a protective factor in cardiovascular disease. The role of oestrogen therapy is important with regard to lipid changes but it is thought unlikely that these changes fully explain the benefits of oestrogen therapy on the cardiovascular system (Whitehead and Godfree, 1992).

Table 3.2   Changes in lipids and lipoproteins after the menopause

Lipid/lipoprotein	Change in concentration
Total cholesterol	↑
Low density lipoprotein (LDL)	↑
High density lipoprotein (HDL)	↓

↑, increase; ↓, decrease.

Clotting factors

Hormone replacement therapy may have a beneficial effect on coagulation and fibrinolysis (Gilligan et al, 1994). Thrombotic effects of the oral contraceptive pill do not necessarily apply to HRT. Further research is needed to establish the effects of HRT on existing clotting disorders.

Vessel walls

Beneficial effects, directly to the blood vessel walls may also be partly responsible for the beneficial effects of oestrogen to the cardiovascular system. Oestrogen has a vasodilatory effect which can produce a reduction in blood pressure, improve arterial blood flow and improve cardiac output (Gilligan et al, 1994; Gangar et al, 1991).

Insulin metabolism

Diabetes is a well known risk factor for heart disease. Pancreatic insulin resistance may be improved by oestrogen therapy, making a contribution to the overall cardiovascular benefits (Godsland et al, 1993; Stevenson et al, 1994).

Body fat distribution

It is recognized that there are two types of body fat distribution. **Android** (or male type) is demonstrated by fat around the abdominal region whereas **Gynoid** (or female type) is demonstrated by more fat around the hips and thighs. The terms 'apple-shaped' or 'pear-shaped' are sometimes used to describe which category a person falls into. Android fat distribution ('apples') is associated with a higher risk of heart disease. The menopause is thought to influence a redistribution of fat toward a male pattern, which may be reversed by HRT (Ley et al, 1992).

Other risk factors for cardiovascular disease

Oestrogen therapy has been widely recommended as a way of reducing cardiovascular risk in postmenopausal women. There are many other factors, however, which will influence a woman's individual risk of developing heart disease. It is important to treat all aspects of a woman's health and not just analyse her hormone or lipid profile. If we are to give full, informed advice, this will mean taking time to assess other factors in relation to diet and lifestyle. There seems little sense in offering a woman HRT if we fail to give advice about other issues which will influence her individual risk of developing cardiovascular problems. Furthermore, some women will find it easier to make positive lifestyle changes in an effort to reduce the risk of heart disease but might not be willing to consider HRT. Ideally we should be encouraging women to consider all influencing factors and how their lifestyle may need to be adjusted accordingly. This advice should include accurate information about the effects of HRT.

Lifestyle factors which increase the risk of cardiovascular disease are:

- Smoking
- Obesity
- Diet
- Lack of regular exercise
- High-fat diet

Women with certain medical conditions may be at particular risk of cardiovascular disease and it could be argued that they should be targetted to receive information about HRT as well as lifestyle advice (see Chapter 8).

Medical risk factors for cardiovascular disease are:

- Hypertension
- Family history of heart disease
- Diabetes
- Hypercholesterolaemia

In the future we may see the results of long-term trials prospectively evaluating the effect of HRT on the cardiovascular system. Such studies would take years to conduct, require a very large number of women and be extremely costly. In the meantime we must advise women according to current medical opinion and ensure that the information we pass on is accurate and up-to-date.

REFERENCES

Argen M, Karrellas A, Leahey D et al (1991) Ultrasound attenuation of the calcaneous in post menopausal women. *Calcif. Tissue Int.* **48**: 240–244.

Barrett-Connor E & Kritz-Silverstein D (1993) Estrogen replacement therapy and cognitive function in older women. *J. Am. Med. Assoc.* **269**: 2637–2641.

Baud CA, Very JM & Corvoisier B (1988) Biophysical studies of bone mineral content in biopsies of osteoporosis patients before and after long term treatment with fluoride. *Bone* **9**: 361–365.

Bush TL, Barratt-Connor E, Cowan LD et al (1987) Cardiovascular mortality and non-contraceptive use of oestrogen in women. Results from the Lipid Research Clinics Program Follow-Up Study. *Circulation* **75**: 1102–1109.

Chow R, Harrison JE & Notarius C (1987) Effects of two randomised exercise programmes on bone mass of healthy post menopausal women. *Br. Med. J.* **295**: 1441–1444.

Christiansen C, Christiansen MS & Transbol I (1981) Bone mass in post menopausal women after withdrawal of oestrogen replacement therapy. *Lancet* **1**: 459–461.

Cohn SH, Abesamis C, Ysmasura S et al (1977) Comparative skeletal mass and radial bone mineral content in black and white women. *Metabolism* **26**: 171–178.

Dawson-Hughes B, Dallal GE, Krall EA et al (1991) A controlled trial of the effect of calcium supplementation on bone density in post menopausal women. *N. Engl. J. Med.* **323**: 878–883.

Dempster D, Shane E, Horbert W & Lindsay R (1986) A simple method for correlative scanning microscopy of human iliac crest biopsies. *Bone and Mineral* **1**: 15–21.

Department of Health (1994) *On the state of the nation*. London: HMSO.

Drinkwater BL, Nilson K, Chesunt CH et al (1984) Bone mineral content of amenorrheic and eumenorrheic athletes. *N. Engl. J. Med.* **311**: 277.

Ettinger B, Genant HK & Cann CE (1985) Long term oestrogen therapy prevents bone loss and fractures. *Ann. Intern. Med.* **102**: 319–324.

Falkeborn M, Persson I, Adami HO et al (1992) The risk of acute myocardial infarction after oestrogen and oestrogen/progestogen replacement. *Br. J. Obstet. Gynaecol.* **99**: 821–828.

Finucane FF, Madans J, Bush T et al (1993) Decreased risk of stroke among post menopausal hormone users: Results from a national cohort. *Arch. Intern. Med.* **153**: 73–79.

Gangar KF, Vyas S, Whitehead MI et al (1991) Pulsatility index in the internal carotid artery in relation to transdermal oestradiol and time since menopause. *Lancet* **338**: 839–842.

Gilligan DM, Badar DM, Panza JA et al (1994) Acute vascular effects of oestrogen in post menopausal women. *Circulation* **90**: 786–791.

Godsland IF et al (1993) Insulin resistance, secretion and elimination in post menopausal women receiving oral or transdermal HRT. *Metabolism* **42**: 846–853.

Gordon T, Kannel WB, Hjortland MC et al (1978) Menopause and coronary heart disease: The Framingham Study. *Ann. Intern. Med.* **89**: 157–161.

Grimley-Evans J (1990) The significance of osteoporosis. In Smith R (ed.) *Osteoporosis*, pp. 1–8. London: Royal College of Physicians.

Grimley-Evans J, Prudham D & Wardles I (1979) A prospective study of fractured femur, incidence and outcome. *Public Health* (London) **93**: 235–241.

Gruber HE, Ivey JC, Baylink DJ et al (1984) Long term calcitonin therapy in post menopausal osteoporosis. *Metabolism* **33**: 295–303.

Heaney RP (1987) The role of nutrition in prevention and management of osteoporosis. *Clin. Obstet. Gynaecol.* **50**: 833–846.

Henderson BE, Paginini-Hill A & Ross RK (1991) Decreased mortality in users of estrogen replacement therapy. *Arch. Intern. Med.* **151**: 75–78.

Hui SL, Slemenda CW & Johnston CC Jnr (1988) Age and bone mass as predictors of fracture in a prospective study. *J. Clin. Invest.* **81**: 1804–1809.

Johnstone CC Jr, Hui SL, Witt RM et al (1985) Early menopausal changes in bone mass and sex steroids. *J. Clin. Endocrinol. Metab.* **61**: 905–911.

Kandlers B, Lindsay R, Dempster DW et al (1984) Determinants of bone mass in young healthy women. In Christiansen (ed.) *Osteoporosis*, pp. 337–340. Aalborg: Stiftsborgtrykken.

Kanis JA & Passmore R (1989) Calcium supplementation of the diet. *Br. Med. J.* **298**: 137–140.

Leichter I, Marguelis JY, Weinrab A et al (1982) The relationship between bone density, bone mineral content and mechanical strength in the femoral neck. *Clin. Orthop.* **163**: 272–281.

Ley CJ, Lees B & Stevenson JC (1992) Sex and menopause-associated changes in body fat distribution. *Am. J. Clin. Nutr.* **55**: 950–954.

Lindsay RL, Hart DM & Clark DM (1978) Bone response to termination of oestrogen treatment. *Lancet* **i**: 1325–1327.

Lobo RA (1991) Clinical Review 27: Effects of hormonal replacement therapy on lipids and lipoproteins in post menopausal women. *J. Clin. Endocrinol. Metab.* **73**: 925–930.

Paginini-Hill A & Henderson VW (1994) Estrogen deficiency and risk of Alzheimer's disease in women. *Am. J. Epidemiol.* **140**: 256–261.

Paginini-Hill A, Ross AK, Gerkins VR et al (1981) Oestrogen therapy use and hip fracture. *Ann. Intern. Med.* **95**: 28–31.

Riggs BL, Wahner HW, Seeman E et al (1982) Changes in bone mineral density of the proximal femur and spine with ageing. Differences between the post menopausal and senile osteoporosis syndromes. *J. Clin. Invest.* **70**: 716–723.

Rosenberg L, Hennekens CH, Rosner B et al (1981) Early menopause and the risk of myocardial infarction. *Am. J. Obstet. Gynaecol.* **139**: 47–51.

Stampfer MJ (1994) Hormone replacement therapy and cardiovascular disease. *Eur. Menopause J.* **1**: 7–8.

Stampfer MJ & Colditz GA (1991) Oestrogen replacement therapy and coronary heart disease: A quantative assessment of the epidemiological evidence. *Prevent. Med.* **20**: 47–63.

Stampfer MJ, Willet WC, Colditz GA et al (1985) A prospective study of post menopausal estrogen therapy and coronary heart disease. *N. Engl. J. Med.* **313**: 1044–1049.

Stevenson JC & Marsh MS (1992) *An Atlas of Osteoporosis* (Encyclopaedia of Visual Medicine Series). Carnforth: Parthenon Publishing Ltd.

Stevenson JC, Lees B, Devonport M et al (1989) Determinants of bone density in normal women: risk factors for future osteoporosis? *Br. Med. J.* **298**: 924–928.

Stevenson JC, Cust MP, Gangar KF et al (1990) Effects of transdermal versus oral HRT on bone mineral density in spine and proximal femur in post menopausal women. *Lancet* **335**: 265–269.

Stevenson JC, Crook D & Godsland IF (1993) Influence of age and menopause on serum lipids and lipoproteins in healthy women. *Atherosclerosis* **98**: 83–90.

Stevenson JC, Crook D, Godsland IF et al (1994) HRT and the cardiovascular system: non lipid effects. *Drugs* **47**(suppl. 2): 35–41.

Sullivan JM, Zwang RV, Hughes JP et al (1990) Estrogen replacement therapy and coronary heart disease. *Arch. Intern. Med.* **150**: 2557–2562.

Wasnich RD, Ross PD, Vogel JM et al (1987) The relative strengths of osteoporosis risk factors in a prospective study of post menopausal osteoporosis. *J. Bone Min. Res.* **2**(suppl. 1): 343.

Whitehead MI & Godfree V (1992) *Hormone Replacement Therapy – Your questions answered*. London: Churchill Livingstone.

Chapter 4

Premature Ovarian Failure

It is most common for the menopause to occur naturally during the late forties or early fifties. Some women however, experience the menopause at a much earlier age, even as young as the late teens or twenties. When the menopause occurs before the age of forty, it is described as **premature**.

Primary ovarian failure occurs when the woman fails to menstruate at all and endocrinological tests reveal ovarian failure. Such women may be very young when the diagnosis is made and it is often associated with genetic disorder.

Secondary ovarian failure arises when a woman has menstruated normally but subsequently experiences amenorrhoea as a result of ovarian failure.

The consequences of an early menopause are greater than with a so-called 'normal' menopause and most specialists would agree that not only do such women deserve particular medical attention, but that they also require a great deal of psychological and emotional support. Society expects women of a certain age to be approaching the 'change of life' and women themselves are mentally prepared for the inevitable. When the ovaries cease to function at a younger age, for whatever reason, or if they are surgically removed, women may feel cheated, that their bodies have let them down and even that they are losing their femininity.

Health professionals working in the field of menopause have a duty to ensure that these women receive adequate medical attention as well as emotional help and support. This chapter defines premature menopause, its causes and effects and discusses the medical management of women experiencing an early menopause. It also outlines some of the emotional and psychological issues which women may need help to deal with at this time.

DEFINITION

Premature ovarian failure is a syndrome occurring prior to the age of forty, characterized by primary or secondary amenorrhoea, elevated gonadotrophic levels and low oestrogen levels (Cohen and Speroff, 1991). Bilateral oophorectomy will also result in a sudden early menopause.

Potential consequences of an early menopause are:

- Vasomotor symptoms
- Psychological symptoms
- Sexual problems
- Infertility
- Osteoporosis
- Arterial disease

INCIDENCE

It is difficult to assess true incidence of early menopause as it is likely that many women will not actually be diagnosed with the condition. Premature ovarian failure accounts for 2–10% of women with primary or secondary amenorrhoea and it is estimated that 1–3% of the general female population is affected (Coulam et al, 1986).

CAUSES

- Surgery
- Iatrogenic
- Natural/spontaneous

Surgery

The most obvious cause of early menopause is removal of the ovaries. Ovaries are usually removed only in the presence of disease, but when they are both removed, menopause is induced. Symptoms may occur within a very short space of time if HRT is not prescribed. Long-term HRT will be necessary for protection of the skeletal and cardiovascular systems. Women who undergo early menopause as a result of surgery are particularly at risk of osteoporosis and heart disease, if left untreated (Richelson et al, 1984; Colditz et al, 1987)

Hysterectomy alone, with conservation of ovaries may also bring forward the expected date of menopause (Siddle et al, 1987). Many women are led to believe that one remaining ovary will continue to function as normal until the expected date of menopause and are not warned that the menopause may occur earlier. Such women may ignore any symptoms suggestive of menopause or be dismissed as being 'too young'. Asymptomatic women may not receive HRT which could be necessary if the menopause occurs early. Some specialists recommend periodic measurements of follicle stimulating hormone to establish onset of menopause in such women.

Iatrogenic

Ovarian failure can be caused by external factors such as:

- Radiotherapy
- Chemotherapy

Radiotherapy

Doses of up to 500 rads cause ovarian failure in 60% of women (Cohen and Speroff, 1991). Doses of 800 rads lead to permanent ovarian failure. Treatment doses for Hodgkin's disease and Lymphoma are usually 4500 rads, although shielding of the ovaries will reduce the amount of radiation reaching the ovaries (Baker et al, 1972).

Chemotherapy

Chemotherapeutic agents will have an adverse effect on ovarian function in most women. Women over 30 years at the time of the chemotherapy are likely to experience permanent ovarian failure, whilst young women are at risk of an earlier menopause, but several years later (Whitehead et al, 1983).

Natural/spontaneous causes

Sometimes the ovaries fail spontaneously, or naturally, but at an unusually early age. Women may present with typical menopausal symptoms or they may be asymptomatic. Diagnosis of premature ovarian failure may result from investigations into a separate condition, such as infertility or prolonged amenorrhoea. In such instances an unexpected diagnosis of early menopause is very traumatic.

A true cause for the early menopause is often never discovered but in some women the following may be the cause:

- Genetic factors
- Metabolic causes
- Autoimmune disease
- Infection

Genetic factors

The majority of women with early menopause have a normal 46XX karyotype (Alper and Garner, 1985), but some women show an abnormality on a specific part of the X chromosome. This is demonstrated by a familial link in some cases. Chromosomal abnormalities are more common in women with primary rather than secondary failure of the ovaries.

Metabolic causes

It has been shown that the development of ovarian failure can be due directly to metabolic disturbances. However, this is a rare cause of early menopause (Cohen and Speroff, 1991).

Autoimmune disease

Some women with premature ovarian failure have a history of autoimmune disease (Perkonen et al, 1986). Blood tests can be performed to establish whether this could be a cause.

Infection

Infections with the mumps virus can cause damage to the ovaries (Morison et al, 1976). Three percent of women with pelvic tuberculosis will develop ovarian failure (Nogales-Ortiz et al, 1979).

Resistant ovary syndrome

Resistant ovary syndrome is thought to be an early stage of ovarian failure (Godfree, 1995). Diagnosis is only definitive following ovarian biopsy, with immature follicles present in the ovaries. Clinical management of resistant ovary syndrome is identical to that of premature ovarian failure (Cohen and Speroff, 1991). Pregnancies have occurred in women with resistant ovary syndrome, but it is not possible to predict a response to therapy, so some would argue that ovarian biopsy is not clinically useful (Godfree, 1995).

CLINICAL ASSESSMENT

It is essential that women suspected of premature ovarian failure are comprehensibly assessed. The diagnosis, once made, may be traumatic and for many women, and will have implications with regard to fertility, feelings of femininity and physical effects. As well as a full physical examination and treatment, **strong psychological support** is essential.

Diagnosis

A diagnosis of premature ovarian failure is considered in women with a history of amenorrhoea, who may or may not be experiencing menopause type symptoms. Measurement of FSH levels are performed serially on at least three occasions. A persistently raised FSH concentration cannot be considered as absolute evidence of ovarian failure, because studies have shown that a few women with levels above 40 IU/l have ovulated and even become pregnant (Rebar et al, 1982); however, this is extremely rare.

Opinion is divided as to whether ovarian biopsies are of clinical value. A biopsy will differentiate between premature ovarian failure (where no follicles will be identified) and resistant ovary syndrome (where immature follicles may be seen). However, clinical management is unlikely to change. There are also the risks associated with general anaesthetic, surgery and postoperative recovery. Postoperative adhesions may also occur, hindering any efforts at assisted conception at a later date.

The diagnosis of premature menopause is always traumatic and can follow several months of clinical investigations. Referral to a specialist centre is advisable so that the necessary tests, investigations and counselling can be carried out as promptly as possible.

TREATMENT

In view of the increased risk of both osteoporosis and heart disease in women with premature ovarian failure, it is essential that women receive adequate oestrogen replacement (combined with progestogen when required). For most women this will mean long-term hormone replacement therapy. It is important that each woman is given the information she needs, to decide with her doctor, which particular form of HRT she will take. There is some evidence that higher than standard doses are required to give adequate relief of symptoms in younger women (Reid and Gangar, 1994). HRT will be recommended until at least the normal age of the menopause.

Women who do not wish to become pregnant should be warned of the very small theoretical risk of pregnancy and advised on suitable contraception methods. Those women who do desire pregnancy will need extensive fertility investigations and counselling, with a view to attempted induction of ovulation or for ovum donation.

PSYCHOLOGICAL SUPPORT

It can be very traumatic for a woman to be told that she is unexpectedly menopausal, particularly if she has yet to have children. It comes as a shock to learn that ovaries have ceased to function and that serious health consequences are possible, if treatment is not considered.

Women often remember vividly the occasion on which they were told the diagnosis of ovarian failure, so it is vital that such information is given as sympathetically as possible. Women speak of being told very abruptly, in busy gynaecological clinics, with little time for discussion or questions. Many women leave the clinic upset, confused and feeling very isolated. They seldom know anyone else with the condition and often do not know where to turn. Blood tests may be performed on several occasions but still the woman is sometimes left feeling unprepared and anxious about the possible diagnosis. At such times any information which is given may not be taken in and remembered.

Support groups are commonly held for women undergoing hysterectomy and women undergoing surgical removal of the ovaries may find help in these groups. Women experiencing spontaneous ovarian failure are often left isolated and anxious. Partners, parents and friends may not be able to offer much help and even from health professionals, there may be little in the way of counselling or psychological support.

In some areas local support groups have been established. The needs of the group will vary according to the age of the women and whether or not they have had children. Women who have completed their families may still experience feelings of grief when confronted with sterility. Women have expressed that the following issues cause anxiety and that opportunity for discussion of them would be helpful:

- Fertility
- Sexuality
- Ageing
- Telling partners/family
- Medical/health consequences, including symptom relief

FERTILITY

Although pregnancies have occurred in women who have been diagnosed with ovarian failure, they are rare and most women wanting children will need extensive fertility management. If reversible ovarian failure is suspected, ovulation induction can be attempted. Otherwise the options are as follows:

- *In vitro* fertilization using ovum donation
- Embryo transfer using ovum donation
- Gamete intra fallopian transfer (GIFT) using ovum donation
- Adoption

In conclusion, the impact of a diagnosis of premature ovarian failure is often underestimated. There is little available in the way of information leaflets, books and videos about the subject. The majority of booklets about menopause assume an age of around 50 years and for the younger woman they are inappropriate. Each woman should therefore be treated individually with as much attention being paid to her nonphysical health as to the physical. At present some women are not even given the information they need to look after their physical health after an early menopause, let alone the psyche and emotions.

REFERENCES

Alper MM & Garner PR (1985) Premature ovarian failure: its relationship to autoimmune disease. *Obstet. Gynaecol.* **66**: 27.

Baker WJ, Morgan RL, Peckham MJ et al (1972) Reservation of ovarian function in patients requiring radiotherapy for para-aortic and pelvic Hodgkin's disease. *Lancet* **ii**: 1307.

Cohen I & Speroff L (1991) Premature ovarian failure: update. *Obstet. Gynaecol. Survey* **46**: 156–161.

Colditz GA, Willett WC, Stampfer MJ et al (1987) Menopause and the risk of coronary heart disease in women. *N. Engl. J. Med.* **316**: 1105.

Coulam CB, Anderson SC & Annegars JF (1986) Incidence of premature ovarian failure. *Obstet. Gynaecol.* **67**: 604.

Coulam CB, Kempers RD & Randel RV (1982) Premature ovarian failure: evidence for the autoimmune mechanisms. *Fertil. Steril.* **36**: 238.

Godfree V (1995) *British Menopause Society Presentation on Premature Ovarian Failure*. June.

Morison JC, Gimes JR, Wiser LW et al (1976) Mumps oophritis: A cause of premature menopause. *Fertil. Steril.* **26**: 255.

Nogales-Ortiz F, Tarancon I & Nogales FF (1979) The pathology of female genital tuberculosis. *Obstet. Gynaecol.* **53**: 422.

Perkonen F, Siegberg R, Makinen T et al (1986) Immunological disturbance in patients with premature ovarian failure. *Clin. Endocrinol.* **25**: 1.

Rebar RW, Erickson GF & Yen SSC (1982) Ideopathic premature ovarian failure: Clinical and endocrine characteristics. *Fertil. Steril.* **37**: 35.

Reid BA & Gangar KF (1994) Premature menopause and HRT: are conventional regimens adequate? *Contemp. Rev. Obstet. Gynaecol.* **6**: 44–45.

Richelson LS, Wahner HW, Melton LJ III et al (1984) Relative contributions of ageing and estrogen deficiency to post menopausal bone loss. *N. Engl. J. Med.* **311**: 1273.

Siddle N, Sarrel P & Whitehead MI (1987) The effects of hysterectomy on the age of ovarian failure: identification of a subgroup of women with premature loss of ovarian function and literature review. *Fertil. Steril.* **47**: 94–100.

Whitehead E, Shiet SM, Blackledge G et al (1983) The effect of combination chemotherapy on ovarian function in women treated for Hodgkin's disease. *Cancer* **52**: 988.

Chapter 5

Women's Perspectives on Menopause

The only consistent factor in every woman's experience of the menopause is that eventually menstruation stops. Other than this, you can help to prepare a woman for the onset of menopause, explaining what might happen and how she may feel, but you cannot say for certain how she *will* feel. Every woman's experience of the climacteric period is unique; her life will be influenced by many factors other than just hormonal ones. Her expectations of the menopause and related symptoms, her life experiences, her culture and her circumstances will all influence her perception and experience of the climacteric.

CHANGING TIMES

Attitudes to the menopause have changed over the years, particularly as society itself has changed (Dickson, 1995).

In the Victorian era, the word menopause would hardly have been mentioned as being of medical concern, except perhaps to recognize that it sometimes resulted in women having a 'nervous disposition'. Women themselves would have welcomed it as a release from childbearing. In the early to mid 20th century, the menopause was viewed as a time of loss or decay. Women were often prescribed tranquillizers or antidepressants, showing that the climacteric was viewed as a time of distress. Now, in the late 20th century, the menopause is sometimes viewed as a deficiency disease which needs to be 'treated', particularly by the medical profession who tend to have 'medicalized' the menopause in some respects. Women may feel that they are less feminine after the menopause, or less healthy, if they decline the offered hormone replacement therapy. Yet women are anxious about the use of HRT and want to be sure that it is really safe and appropriate before they consider its use.

As we move towards the 21st century, stereotypes are being recast – women are no longer considered 'over the hill' at 50, but rather may experience what has been termed a 'post-menopausal zest' (Sheehy, 1993).

If 45 is the old age of youth, 50 is the youth of a woman's second adulthood
(Gail Sheehy, *The Silent Passage.*)

The menopause is no longer a sickness but a 'transition phase' into a new life. Women are seeking information on the subject of menopause and want to decide for themselves whether or not to take HRT. The media play an important role in informing women about the menopause and HRT. This has both positive and negative implications for women's knowledge about the subject. One thing is certain however, women no longer consider the menopause as a taboo subject – they actively seek the information they need to be informed. Armed with the facts, gleaned from women's magazines, radio chat shows and television documentaries, they resent medics trying to make the decision for them about HRT. Women want to be accurately informed and actively involved in the decision as to whether to take HRT. Women are also turning to alternative means of alleviating menopausal symptoms using complementary or nonhormonal therapies. The modern challenge to women is to 'know your own menopause' or as Gail Sheehy puts it in her book, *The Silent Passage* – 'claim the pause'.

CHANGING CULTURES

The menopause is inevitable for those women who live long enough, but how it is experienced is unique to individuals. Even purely physiological symptoms such as hot flushes, sweats and vaginal dryness are not universally experienced, or at least acknowledged, by all cultures. Lock, studying Japanese women and Wright studying Navaho Indians, found that in each of these cultures, there are no words for 'hot flush' (Wright, 1983; Lock, 1991). Symptom reporting in Japan is significantly lower than in women from North America (Lock, 1994). Lock reminds us, though, that when considered alongside Japan's low incidence of heart disease, breast cancer and its high life expectancy it is possible that biological factors as well as psychological ones will influence their experience of menopausal symptoms.

For some African women the time of menopause indicates a higher social status and life becomes easier after it. This means that the menopause is seen as a positive life event, whereas in countries such as the USA, Germany and Italy, the menopause is viewed in a negative way – as a demarcation of ageing (Flint, 1994). This may influence how a woman feels at the time of the menopause.

In China, few women seek advice about the menopause, although it is possible that women do experience symptoms, but suffer in silence. Chinese women generally perceive the menopause as a natural process and so perhaps have a positive attitude towards any symptoms they may experience (Tang, 1994).

In the UK, cultural differences are less profound but still important, particularly with regard to the use of hormone replacement therapy. The following factors are worth considering:

- Catholic women may associate HRT with the contraceptive pill and refuse it because of religious objections. Careful counselling on the differences between HRT and the contraceptive pill are required.

• Orthodox Jews or Muslim women may not wish to resume bleeding again after the menopause because of religious restrictions during menstruation. HRT regimens which achieve amenorrhoea may be acceptable.

• Vegetarians or vegans may be keen to know whether their HRT is derived directly from animals. Alternatives, derived from plants, may be preferred.

CHANGING PRESSURES

The climacteric is a time in a woman's life of great physical change, which may last months or even years. For the average woman, these hormonal changes will occur at around the age of 50 years when she may also be experiencing pressures in other areas of her life. All of these other factors may influence how a woman feels and also how she copes with any menopausal symptoms which may occur. Longstanding problems may become harder to live with or to deal with when a woman is also experiencing physical or psychological upset as a result of hormonal changes. Every woman approaching the menopause has a variety of needs, not just hormonal ones so it is important to take a holistic approach and consider all aspects of a woman's life, not simply her hormones.

'It's your age'

There is a tendency to blame the menopause for every upset or complaint which arises around this time of a woman's life. Anxiety, depression, panic attacks may all be labelled as being menopausal symptoms and for some women it can be hard to simply find a listening ear. Certainly the menopause cannot be blamed for every emotional upset, although some problems may be exacerbated by hormonal influences, causing longstanding problems to be highlighted or new ones to be recognized.

Factors which may affect a woman's attitudes to the menopause include:

- Changing body image
- Ageing
- Attitudes towards sexuality
- Dreams/expectations
- Relationships
- 'Empty nest' syndrome
- Roles/responsibilities

Changing body image

The media would have use believe that all women should be slim to be beautiful. Society strives towards maintaining a youthful figure into middle age and beyond. Large sums of money are spent by women trying to lose weight and keep young looking. Yet it is a fact of life that as we get older, our bodies do change and unless one can afford plastic surgery, it is inevitable that we will begin to 'show our age'. Wrinkles may appear, hair often greys, waistlines thicken and muscles sag, particularly if underused. Both men and women have to grow to accept their changing bodies and yet still look after them. HRT is not a youth drug and will not prevent many of the effects of ageing on the body. Exercise, diet and lifestyle are probably more important factors (see Chapter 8). Women who turn to HRT hoping to 'turn back the clock' will be sadly disappointed.

Ageing

The menopause is an event most women cannot ignore. Some women see the menopause as marking the beginning of new freedom, new choices and new challenges. For others it represents a turning point, a stage in life one step nearer to old age and, ultimately, death. Attitudes to ageing vary, but for some women, the menopause may be an uncomfortable reminder of one's lost youth and vigour. For those women who struggle with acute menopausal symptoms, the perimenopausal phase may be a difficult one to come to terms with, as they wonder how long these symptoms really will continue.

An understanding of a woman's perspective will help when trying to counsel or advise a woman at this time.

Sexuality

The menopause marks the end of the fertile years. Contraception can (eventually) be stopped and sexual intercourse continued without concern about pregnancy. For some, this is a release, for others a sadness, perhaps highlighting the ageing process. A woman may feel less desirable or less attractive to her partner. This along with physical effects such as vaginal dryness or reduced libido, may lead to sexual difficulties at this time. Sensitive counselling, practical advice, HRT if appropriate and sometimes psychosexual therapy, will be of benefit.

Dreams/expectations

Some women look upon the menopause as a life event, a stage in life to be recognized and coped with, either in a positive way or negatively. It may be a time of evaluation of past life or of planning for a future one. Women may look back with regret because of failed dreams or sad memories. For childless women, the menopause, marking the end of the reproductive era, may be particularly poignant.

For working women, success may not be as great as one had hoped, promotion may be out of reach and retirement becomes the next major step. Marriages and relationships may come under scrutiny, particularly as children leave home and women are given more time to evaluate their own lives. Expectations of life may not be fulfilled, the partner may be going through similar 'mid life' thoughts and decisions. Some women may feel as though the menopause is simply highlighting negative aspects of life, rather than signifying a time of new beginnings and expectations. Helping a woman to understand both the negatives and the positives of middle age may help her deal more easily with the hormonal effects of the menopause.

Relationships

Mid life can be a time when relationships are tested or re-evaluated. Marriages may be faltering and need a concerted effort to revive them. Physical and psychological effects of the menopause can test a stable, loving relationship, yet alone one which is faltering. Men too, may be experiencing difficulties, as they come to terms with approaching middle age. Men do not experience a true hormonal change in the same way as women do, but they undoubtedly have to face similar issues regarding health, work and sexuality. Couples may seek help in making adjustments to changing roles and changing lives. For some couples, relationship counselling may be of benefit.

'Empty nest' syndrome

The so called 'empty nest' syndrome is used to describe the feelings of sadness and emptiness which a woman may experience when her last child leaves home. A woman who has dedicated her whole life to the upbringing of her children may struggle with the new role she finds herself in – as an independent woman and/or partner. In these days when many women work outside the home and are encouraged to pursue personal interests as well as those of her family, these feelings may be less intense.

Roles and responsibilities

Mid life may be viewed as a time of increased freedom – children leaving home, finances may be more secure, work life may be settled. It can come as a shock to some to realize that just as they are losing the dependence of their children, their own parents may be coming more dependent on them. Women may find themselves torn between caring for their parents and remaining loyal to their partner. For some this may lead to feelings of resentment and frustration, leading to guilt when the elderly parent does die. Counselling may be of help in these circumstances.

Some women also struggle with the changing roles from mother to grandmother, as their own children have families of their own. Yet the role of grandparent can be immensely satisfying and rewarding.

Work relationships may change. For most women, menopausal symptoms are not usually severe enough to require more than simple adaptations to the working life, such as opening more windows, wearing layers of clothes and keeping a notebook for those forgotten messages! However, those women who do lose their job during mid life, for whatever reason, may find it very difficult to get back into the workplace. A woman may find that her husband is reaching the peak of his career, with all its satisfaction and achievements, just at the point that she feels unsettled in work or poorly motivated, because of climacteric symptoms.

When advising a woman about the menopause and hormone replacement therapy, try and find what other factors, socially, emotionally or physically, may be affect ing how she feels. Helping her to cope with some of these other difficulties may make it easier for her to cope with the menopause. Alternatively, helping her through the hormonal upset of the menopause, may make her more able to cope with other problems by herself.

CONTRACEPTION AT THE PERIMENOPAUSE

The menopause marks the end of a woman's reproductive life, but can only be recognized as such retrospectively. Menstruation may occur after several months of amenor-rhoea, when a woman believed herself to be infertile. Fertility declines appreciably once a women is in her forties (Spira, 1988) and frequency of intercourse lessens in many instances (Trussell and Westoff, 1980). Pregnancy is therefore unusual but not impossible. It is important to remember that in 1990 there were over 400 termina-tions of pregnancy in women over the age of 45 years in England and Wales (OPCS, 1991).

Pregnancy in a woman over the age of 45 years is known to be high risk, with 25% of pregnancies ending in miscarriage (Wilson, 1992). Similarly, maternal and perinatal mortality rates are significantly higher in older women (Guillebaud, 1985). There is also a greater risk of a baby being born with congenital abnormalities such as Down's syndrome. Along with the physical problems associated with a pregnancy at this time, psychological and emotional difficulties may accompany what is often an unwanted pregnancy.

It is therefore crucial that women are warned of the continuing need for contraception during the perimenopause. Many women wrongly believe that they are infertile during this time or 'take a chance' that they will not be the one to fall pregnant.

How long is contraception necessary?

The Family Planning Association recommendations are that women under the age of 50 should continue using contraception until they have experienced 2 years of amenorrhoea. Over the age of 50, women should continue using contraception for at least 1 year after their last period. For women not on HRT, these recommendation are simple if a little tedious. Women may feel that one of the few advantages of menopause is that contraception becomes (eventually) unnecessary. To have to continue using contraception for 12–24 months can seem an unnecessary precaution, but most women do not want to run the risk of pregnancy.

Once a perimenopausal woman starts on HRT, it becomes much more difficult to advise about when to stop using contraception. Bleeding may continue with the use of HRT and even if amenorrhoea occurs, a woman cannot assume that she is infertile. Theoretically, you could ask a woman to stop HRT and measure levels of follicle stimulating hormone 6–8 weeks later. If raised, this would indicate menopause. However, in practice, most women do not want to stop HRT for this reason alone and in any case you could still not absolutely guarantee that pregnancy would not occur (Metcalf and Donald, 1979).

It is therefore impossible to give absolute recommendations as to when a woman on HRT can stop using contraception. In practice an arbitrary figure of around

54 years is suggested, although it should be stressed to women that this is only a guide. Each woman will make her own decision based on her perception and acceptance of risk, which will be influenced by the following:

- Age
- Frequency of coitus
- How easily she previously became pregnant
- Male fertility (younger man may be more fertile)
- Acceptibility of methods of contraception

Combined oral contraception

The combined contraceptive pill can be used by a woman during the perimenopausal phase providing that the following criteria are met:

- She is a non-smoker
- She is normotensive
- She is not obese
- She has no family history of cardiovascular disease and no cardiovascular risk factors

In the light of recommendations from the Committee on Safety of Medicines 1995 following preliminary studies showing an increased risk of thrombosis with pills containing desogestrel or gestodene (Spitzer et al, 1996), it is particularly important that any risk of cardiovascular disease is eliminated before allowing a perimenopausal woman to continue the combined pill. Women must be involved in a frank discussion regarding the risks and benefits of continuing its use until the time of the menopause.

Effect on the menopause

Use of the combined pill will cause menopausal symptoms to be masked, as oestrogen levels remain high as a result of the pill. The oestrogen will also offer protection against osteoporosis. The exact time of the last period will not be known as regular withdrawal bleeds are likely to continue.

The progestogen-only pill

The progestogen only pill (POP) or 'mini pill' can safely be taken during the perimenopause. It works in the following ways:

- Changes quality of cervical mucus
- Renders the endometrium unreceptive to a fertilized oocyte so implantation cannot occur
- Affects the mobility of the Fallopian tubes, preventing spermatozoa from travelling to meet an ovum.

Although the rate of pregnancy in women using the POP is often quoted as 1–4 pregnancies per 100 woman years, the rate among older women users is the most favourable (Bisset et al, 1990; Vessey et al, 1990).

Effect on the menopause

Use of the POP will not usually mask the onset of menopausal symptoms. Amenorrhoea may occur with the use of the POP and women may wonder whether the menopause has occurred. If a woman does experience prolonged amenorrhoea on the POP, she cannot assume she is becoming postmenopausal. Serial FSH measurements are not affected by the use of the POP. Some doctors recommend the use of the POP alongside oestrogen as a form of both HRT and contraception, although this particular regimen has not been subjected to clinical trials for contraceptive efficacy. Theoretically it seems logical.

Injectable and implanted progestogens

One of the main drawbacks of these methods, when considering use in perimenopausal women, is the fact that they are longlasting. Most women at this time are looking for contraception which is convenient to use, but also easy to stop after the menopause. They are extremely reliable forms of contraception but can cause irregular bleeding and side-effects such as weight gain and mood swings. It would be difficult to consider the use of

HRT alongside such methods, because of the risk of irregular bleeding.

Intrauterine systems (IUS)

Modern IUS offer a very satisfactory form of contraception for women approaching the menopause. They are longlasting and have few side-effects. A device inserted at the age of 40 years is unlikely to be replaced unless the woman experiences problems. It will be left *in situ* and removed after the menopause. The woman then has adequate contraceptive cover throughout the perimenopausal era.

An IUS containing levonorgestrel is available (Fig. 5.1). For perimenopausal women it has the advantage of suppressing endometrial response and in many instances producing amenorrhoea. It is licensed for contraceptive use in the UK, but could also be used in conjunction with oestrogen as a form of HRT (Anderson et al, 1992; Raudaskoski et al, 1995).

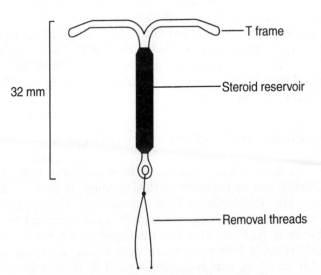

Figure 5.1   Levonorgestrel releasing intrauterine system.

Barrier Methods

- Condom – male and female
- Diaphragm
- Spermicidal pessaries
- Spermicidal foam

Barrier methods of contraception (Fig. 5.2) are commonly used by women at around the time of the menopause. They have no effect on hormonal changes and so will not influence the onset of menopause or mask symptoms at this time. They are easily stopped when contraception is no longer required.

Learning how to use a method such as a condom or cap can be difficult for a woman who has never used this method before, particularly if she is beginning to suffer vaginal dryness as a result of oestrogen deficiency. However a couple who are used to such methods may find them convenient to continue through the climacteric years.

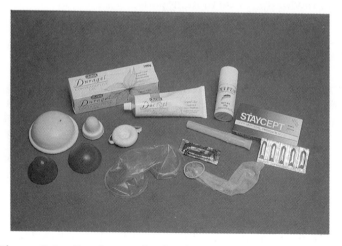

Figure 5.2   Barrier methods of contraception. (Courtesy of the Medical Illustration Department, Northwick Park Institute for Medical Research, Northwick Park Hospital, Harrow, Middlesex.)

WOMEN'S PERSPECTIVE ON MENOPAUSE – Contraception at the perimenopause

The decline in fertility in the year leading up to the time of the menopause, means that methods which might be considered unreliable for younger women, probably offer sufficient contraceptive protection to perimenopausal women. This includes the use of spermicidal agents on their own.

The spread of human immunodeficiency virus (HIV) and the subsequent health awareness campaigns, have resulted in barrier methods becoming more popular, particularly with younger women who have grown up with the 'AIDS message'. With an increasing number of women entering new relationships later in life, it could be argued that so-called 'safe sex' should be practised at all ages, including the perimenopause.

Sterilization

It has been estimated that 40% of women aged 40–4 years report that one or other partner has been sterilized (OPCS, 1989) This obviously takes care of the problem of contraception through the perimenopausal years. It is unlikely that sterilization would be considered by a woman who was close to menopause.

Natural methods

A 'natural' approach to contraception appeals to many women. Sexual intercourse is avoided during the fertile time of the cycle, which is recognized by one or more of the following factors:

- Changes in the cervix
- Changes in cervical mucus secretions
- Basal body temperature
- Calendar method

The perimenopause would be a difficult time to learn such methods, because of a woman's changing body at this time. However a woman who is familiar with the method and is aware of changes in her body may be able to rely on the method throughout the perimenopause.

Postcoital or 'emergency' contraception

The combined oestrogen pill regimen can safely be used by perimenopausal women, if there are no contraindications to the general use of oestrogen (Harper, 1995). If the risk of pregnancy is considered to be high, but the woman is unable to take oestrogen therapy, insertion of an IUS may be considered.

REFERENCES

Anderson K, Matteson LA, Rybo G et al (1992) Intrauterine release of levonorgestrel – a new way of adding progestogen in hormone replacement therapy. *Obstet. Gynaecol.* **79**: 963–967.

Bisset AM, Dingwall-Fordyce I & Hamilton MK (1990) The efficacy of the progestogen only pill as a contraceptive method. *Br. J. Family Planning* **16**: 84–87.

Committee on Safety of Medicines (1995) *Combined Oral Contraceptives and Thromboembolism* (letter) London: CSM.

Dickson GL (1995) *Paradigms of menopause: Towards women's perspectives*. North American Menopause Society presentation.

Flint M (1994) Menopause – The global aspect. In *The modern management of the menopause* (Proceedings of the VII International Congress on Menopause 1993). Carnforth: Parthenon Publishing.

Guillebaud J (1985) Contraception for the older woman. *J. Obstet. Gynaecol.* **5**(suppl. 2): 70–77.

Harper C (1995) Contraception in the perimenopause. In Bromham D (ed.) *Contraception*. Sutton, UK: Reed Healthcare Communications.

Lock M (1991) Contested meanings of the menopause. *Lancet* **337**: 1270–1272.

Lock M (1994) Menopause in a cultural setting. *Exp. Geront.* **29(3–4)**: 307–317.

Metcalf MG & Donald RA (1979) Fluctuating ovarian function in perimenopausal women. *NZ Med. J.* **89**: 45.

Office of Population Census and Surveys (1989) General Household Survey 1987. London: HMSO.

Office of Population Census and Surveys (1991) Abortion Statistics 1990, England and Wales. London: HMSO.

Raudaskoski TH, Lahti EI, Kauppila AJ et al (1995) Transdermal estrogen with a levonorgestrel releasing IUD for climacteric complaints: clinical and endometrial responses. *Am. J. Obstet. Gynaecol.* **172**: 114–119.

Sheehy G (1993) *The Silent Passage*. London: Harper Collins.

Spira A (1988) The decline in fertility with age. *Maturitas* **1**: 15.

Spitzer WO, Lewis M, Heinemann LAJ et al (1996) Third generation oral contraceptives and risk of thromboembolic disorders: an international case control study. *Br. Med. J.* 312: 83–88.

Tang G (1994) Menopause –the situation in Hong Kong Chinese women. In *The Modern Management of the Menopause.* Proceedings of the VII International Congress on Menopause, 1993. Carnforth: Parthenon Publishing.

Trussell J & Westoff CF (1980) Contraceptive practice and trends in coital frequency. *Family Planning Perspectives* 12: 246.

Vessey MP, Villard-Mackintosh L & Yeates D (1990) Effectiveness of progestogen only oral contraceptives (letter). *Br. J. Family Planning* 16: 79.

Wilson RCD (1992) *Understanding HRT and the Menopause.* London: Consumer's Association.

Wright AL (1983) A cross-cultural comparison of menopausal symptoms. *Med. Anthropol.* 7: 20–35.

Chapter 6

Principles of Hormone Replacement Therapy

Women approaching their fifties today are facing decisions which were not considered by a previous generation: whether or not to take hormone replacement therapy; whether to take it for relief of menopausal symptoms, or for the longer-term benefits to the skeletal and cardiovascular systems.

The media and, in particular, women's magazines, frequently publish articles about the menopause and HRT. Unfortunately they are not always balanced or accurate and women are often left feeling even more confused about the subject. The decision to take HRT is not always a simple one and some women find it difficult to find the information they need to make an informed choice.

Health professionals too are not always up-to-date. HRT is a rapidly changing field – more and more products are reaching the market place and more and more research is being performed to establish risks and benefits so that women can be confident in the treatment they are offered. This chapter is intended to given an overview of HRT: what it is, risks and benefits, contraindications and side-effects, and reviews the various methods of giving HRT.

WHAT IS HRT?

HRT usually consists of the two hormones, oestrogen and progestogen. It is the oestrogen which reportedly confers benefits to heart and bone and which effectively relieves acute menopausal symptoms. Women who have had a hysterectomy can safely take oestrogen on its own but women with a uterus are generally prescribed both hormones, as oestrogen alone has been demonstrated to increase the likelihood of endometrial hyperplasia (Henderson, 1989). Adding a progestogen prevents this build up of the endometrium and thus reduces the risk of endometrial carcinoma (Whitehead et al, 1990).

Oestrogens used in HRT are **natural** rather than **synthetic**. 17β-Oestradiol, oestrone and oestriol are all types of natural oestrogen used in HRT. When given as HRT, levels of oestrogen in the blood rise to levels similar to a premenopausal level. HRT also prevents the fluctuation of oestrogen levels which are common around the time of the menopause and which often give rise to acute menopausal symptoms. Synthetic oestrogens such as those used in the contraceptive pill, e.g. ethinyloestradiol, are

Table 6.1   Types of oestrogen

Natural	Synthetic
17β-Oestradiol	Ethinyloestradiol
Oestradiol valerate	Mestranol
Oestrone piperazine sulphate	Diethylstilboestrol
Oestriol	Dienoestrol

not used in modern forms of HRT because of the increased risk of thrombosis and hypertension (Upton, 1988). Conjugated oestrogens are used in some forms of HRT. These act in a similar way to natural oestrogens and are therefore classified as natural (Stern, 1982).

In clinical practice there is little difference between the natural oestrogens, all of which appear to be equally effective (Mashchak et al, 1982). No one form of natural oestrogen is better than another although individual women may prefer one to another. The aim of HRT is to provide a level of circulating oestrogen which is sufficient to relieve symptoms and also protect against cardiovascular disease and osteoporosis. For most women this is achieved by standard doses of HRT.

HRT REGIMENS

Oestrogen therapy can be given cyclically or continuously. It is most common for oestrogen to be given on a continuous basis in order to maintain blood levels and to prevent symptoms returning. In the UK, most preparations provide continuous oestrogen therapy. Progestogen can be given cyclically, continuously or tricyclically (Fig. 6.1).

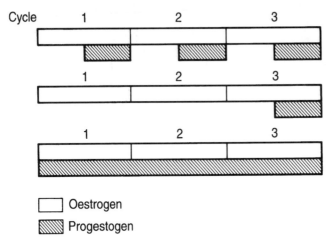

Figure 6.1 **Regimens of oestrogen and progestogen in HRT.**

PRINCIPLES OF HRT
– What is HRT?
– HRT regimens

ROUTES OF ADMINISTRATION

HRT can be given in various ways. There is no ideal way of giving HRT and for many women, the final choice should be an individual one, made in consultation with the supervising doctor. Occasionally there will be medical reasons for choosing one method over another, but in many instances the decision should reflect that treatment which the individual woman is likely to use and which is therefore most likely to be effective (Table 6.2).

Whichever method of giving oestrogen is chosen (except local vaginal treatment), the effect on the uterus is the same, so women with a uterus should be given progestogen as well.

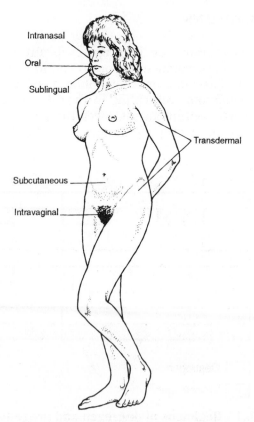

Figure 6.2   Potential routes of oestrogen administration.

Table 6.2 Routes of HRT administration

Oestrogen	Progestogen
Tablet	Tablet
Patch	Patch
Gel	(IUS – not licensed for HRT)
Implant	
Vaginal treatments	

The first pass effect

The main difference between oral and non-oral routes of HRT is the avoidance of the 'first pass' effects on the liver with non-oral routes. Oestradiol given by tablet will pass through both the gut and the liver, resulting in a substantial part being converted into a less potent hormone (Lievertz, 1987). There is wide variation in the rate of absorption between individuals and so the dose requirement for individual women will vary.

Theoretically the first pass effect could produce unwanted changes in the liver, whether such changes are

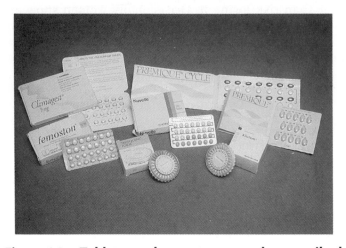

Figure 6.3 Tablets are the most commonly prescribed type of HRT. (Courtesy of the Medical Illustration Department, Northwick Park Institute for Medical Research, Northwick Park Hospital, Harrow, Middlesex.)

clinically relevant to most women is unclear (Whitehead and Godfree, 1992).

Tablets

Tables are a common way of taking HRT and have been available longer than any other method. They are available in varying doses and in combination with a variety of progestogens. Some are conveniently packaged for easy compliance, whilst others can be tailored to an individual's requirements.

Patches

Patches containing oestradiol deliver a constant dose over 24 hours and are changed once or twice weekly. There are two basic types of patch: the reservoir and the matrix patch.

Patches are worn on the buttocks or abdomen and are generally kept in place during swimming and bathing. Reservoir patches stick less well and some women find it easier to remove the patch before swimming or bathing rather than risk losing it. Occasionally women show an allergic reaction to the patch, developing a redness and irritation under the patch, which often persists even after the patch is removed. Matrix patches seem to cause

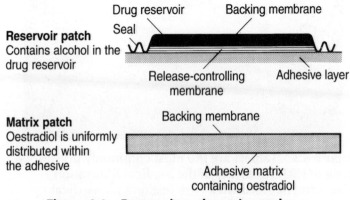

Figure 6.4   Reservoir and matrix patches.

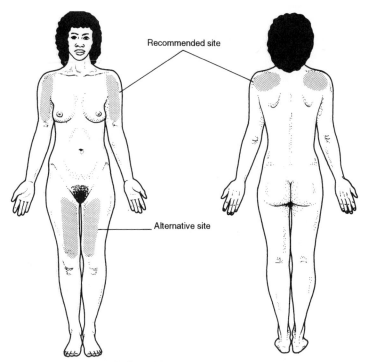

Recommended site

Alternative site

Figure 6.5   Gel should be applied widely and thinly.

less irritation. Women who are allergic to reservoir patches may not be allergic to matrix ones.

Most patches contain only oestrogen but there is an oestrogen/progestogen combination patch, avoiding the need for tablets at all. Patches are also available in compliance kits containing progestogen tablets for nonhysterectomized women.

Gel

An oestradiol-containing gel is available which is gently rubbed into the skin on a daily basis. It should preferably be applied to the upper arms or shoulders. The gel is administered in a measured dose from a pressurized canister. Women should be encouraged to apply the gel over a wide area for maximum absorption. If a woman has not had a hysterectomy, progestogen tablets need to be added to the regimen.

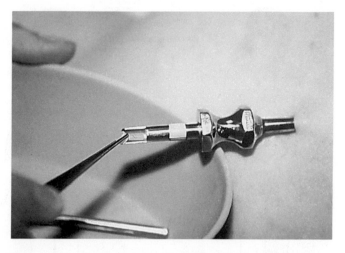

Figure 6.6   Oestrogen or testosterone implantation.

Implants

Oestradiol implants are small pellets which are inserted under the skin of the buttock or abdomen, through a small incision. The oestrogen is then released slowly over a period of months. Generally the higher the implant dose, the longer it will remain effective. Levels of oestrogen in the blood are often higher than with other routes. The hormone testosterone can also be administered by implant, either at the same time as an oestrogen implant or on its own.

There is a wide variation among women as to how long an implant will remain effective. Occasionally the physiological effect of an implant may last up to 2 years so it is important to continue the progestogen therapy in non-hysterectomized women (Whitehead et al, 1993). Rarely, a condition called **tachyphylaxis** may occur, where women return for implants at increasingly shorter intervals (Gangar et al, 1989). Such women experience symptoms even though their oestradiol levels are raised. Repeated implants cause the levels to rise even further. So far it is unclear whether this is harmful, but some specialists would advise caution and withhold implants if oestradiol levels were very high.

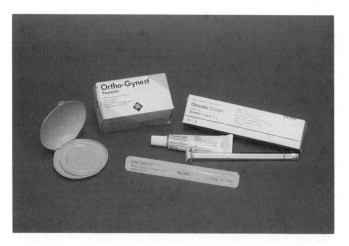

Figure 6.7   Local treatments for vaginal symptoms. (Courtesy of the Medical Illustration Department, Northwick Park Institute for Medical Research, Northwick Park Hospital, Harrow, Middlesex.)

Vaginal treatments

Oestrogen can be administered directly to the vagina by creams, pessaries, tablets and slow-releasing rings. They exert a direct beneficial effect on atrophic vaginitis without systemic effects. They are particularly useful in older women, who need relief of vaginal symptoms but who are reluctant to try systemic HRT.

The oestrogens used in modern vaginal preparations are oestriol and oestradiol. When given at the recommended doses, they are not sufficiently absorbed systemically to cause endometrial proliferation. Prolonged use may lead to an endometrial effect. Vaginal oestrogens should not be used as a lubricant during sexual intercourse because of the small risk of absorption by the male partner.

Intrauterine systems

A progestogen-containing IUS is available for contraceptive purposes. Research is underway looking at its use as an adjunct to oestrogen therapy as a form of hormone replacement. Such a combination may provide endometrium protection without systemic side-effects and for many women, no bleed.

PROGESTOGENS

Progestogens are added to the treatment regimen of non-hysterectomized women in order to prevent endometrial hyperplasia (Persson et al, 1989). Of women taking oestrogen-only therapy, 7–15% will develop endometrial hyperplasia (Sturdee et al, 1978), causing irregular bleeding and the potential to change to endometrial carcinoma (Silverberg, 1988). Adding a progestogen reduces the incidence of irregular bleeding and reduces the risk of endometrial cancer to below that seen in untreated women (Whitehead et al, 1990). Progestogens used in HRT regimens are:

- Norethisterone ⎫
- Levonorgestrel ⎬ Testosterone derived
- Dydrogesterone ⎫
- Medroxyprogesterone acetate ⎬ Progesterone derived

If a women experiences side-effects with a progestogen it is often worth trying one from the other group, which may not have the same effect.

Cyclical progestogens

Progestogens can be given for 10–14 days a cycle in order to prevent endometrial stimulation. Duration of progestogen seems to be as important as dose, with 10 days being the minimum generally recommended in standard doses (Whitehead and Godfree, 1992). Although it is common for progestogens to be prescribed cyclically (i.e. every 28 days), it is sometimes more convenient for a woman to take her progestogen on a calendar month basis (i.e. a 30/31 day 'cycle'). In this instance she would take the progestogen for the first 10 to 14 days of each calendar month. This is much easier to remember than having to count a 28-day cycle. Cyclical progestogen results in a monthly bleed in 80–90% of women.

Doses of progestogen used in cyclical HRT are:

- Norethisterone   1–2.5 mg
- Dydrogesterone   10–20 mg
- Medoxyprogesterone acetate   5–10 mg
- Levonorgestrel   150 μg

Continuous progestogen

A continuous low dose of progestogen alongside continuous oestrogen will prevent hyperplastic changes to the endometrium without the need for a regular bleed (Magos et al, 1985; Archer et al, 1994). This form of therapy is only suitable for truly postmenopausal women (i.e. at least 1 year after the last menstrual bleed) because of the unacceptably high risk of irregular bleeding in perimenopausal women. In any case, irregular bleeding is common in the first few months of therapy and women should be advised of this. If they are able to persevere with the treatment they have a good chance of eventually experiencing amenorrhoea. Continuous oestrogen/progestogen regimens are available or can be tailor-made with a combination of regimens.

Tricyclical progestogens

HRT is also administered in a regimen in which progestogen is given only every 3 months, whilst still maintaining endometrial protection (Ettinger et al, 1994). This results in a bleed once every 3 months which is apparently no heavier than a normal period (Hirvonen et al, 1995). The advantage of this treatment (apart from fewer bleeds) is that potential side-effects of the progestogen are also minimized. For those women who seem unable to tolerate progestogen this is a real advantage.

Progestogen-only therapy

Women who cannot take HRT or who prefer not to, are sometimes prescribed progestogen only to try and alleviate vasomotor symptoms. It is not as effective as oestrogen therapy but may certainly be helpful for some women. Doses of progestogen may need to be higher than those usually given for endometrial protection.

Tibolone

Tibolone is a synthetic type of HRT with oestrogenic, progestogenic and androgenic properties. It is given continuously and does not usually cause bleeding (Rymer, 1992). It is effective at reducing flushes and sweats and improves mood and libido (Benedek-Jaszmann, 1987). It also protects against postmenopausal bone loss. Irregular bleeding may occur in perimenopausal women so it is only recommended for use in postmenopausal women (i.e. at least one year after the last period).

SIDE-EFFECTS OF HRT

Side-effects are common in the first few weeks of starting HRT (Table 6.3). Oestrogen-related side-effects such as breast tenderness, nausea and leg cramps usually subside after 6–8 weeks on therapy. If they do not, a change in dose or type of oestrogen may be necessary.

Progestogen-related side-effects seem to be more common in cyclical regimens and often appear to be similar in type to premenstrual symptoms, e.g. irritability, anxiety, bloatedness and breast pain. They can be minimized by adjusting the dose or type of progestogen whilst ensuring that the minimum dose recommended for endometrial safety is maintained (Siddle, 1989). For more information about management of side-effects see Chapter 7.

Table 6.3   Common side-effects of hormone replacement therapy

Breast tenderness	
Nausea	
Headaches	Often oestrogen-related and transient
Leg cramps	
'PMT'-type symptoms, e.g.	
irritability, bloating, headaches	Often related to progestogen
Irregular bleeding	

BLEEDING PATTERNS AND HRT

Cyclical HRT

Approximately 80–90% of women who use a cyclical form of HRT will experience a monthly bleed. This bleed should be regular, usually lasting between 2 and 6 days and should not be unacceptably heavy. Mild period type pains are common. The first few months on treatment may not produce a regular bleed but after about three cycles the bleed should settle into a regular and predictable pattern.

Monitoring of the withdrawal bleed should take place at follow-up visits to ensure that the pattern is as expected for the regimen being prescribed. When the progestogen is given for 10 or 12 days a month the bleed should occur towards the end of the progestogen course or shortly after. Early bleeding may be a sign that a dose adjustment is required (see Chapter 7 for monitoring of HRT).

Breakthrough bleeding

Breakthrough bleeding, i.e. bleeding unrelated to the progestogen course, should not occur with cyclical forms of HRT. Repeated episodes of breakthrough bleeding will need investigating. Occasional 'one off' episodes may occur due to the following factors:

- Poor compliance (particularly with the progestogen)

- Drug interactions, e.g. antibiotics
- Gastrointestinal upset, leading to poor absorption of the HRT
- Stress occasionally provokes bleeding, although this may be due to unintentionally missing tablets.

See Chapter 7 for management of breakthrough bleeding during use of HRT.

Continuous combined oestrogen and progestogen regimens

The aim of a continuous combined oestrogen/progestogen regimen is to avoid the need for a monthly bleed whilst maintaining endometrial safety. Some women find the thought of returning to monthly bleeds unpleasant so the idea of a 'period-free' HRT is attractive. This is particularly true for older women starting HRT for the first time, many years after their periods have stopped. A postmenopausal woman has a 70% chance of achieving amenorrhoea after an initial 'settling-in' phase, during which spotting is common. Women changing from a cyclical to a continuous regimen should make the change at the end of a withdrawal bleed. Bleeding which occurs during the initial few months of treatment does not need investigating, but prolonged or unacceptable bleeding may require a change of treatment. If bleeding is persistent, clinical investigation will be necessary (D Mackay-Hart, British Menopause Society presentation, 1995).

CONTRAINDICATIONS TO HRT

Much confusion surrounds the issue of true contraindications to HRT. In the past, both medical professionals and the lay public have wrongly applied data relating to the oral contraceptive pill to HRT. This has led to confusion over who can and cannot take HRT safely. Contraindications can be divided into those conditions which usually lead to a woman being advised not to take HRT and those which will warrant further tests or investigations before HRT is prescribed.

Contraindications to HRT are:

- Oestrogen-dependent tumours (e.g. breast/endometrium)
- Undiagnosed abnormal vaginal bleeding
- Pregnancy
- Severe active liver disease
- Otosclerosis

(Whitehead and Godfree, 1992).

Oestrogen-dependent tumours

A recent history of breast cancer or endometrial cancer is generally considered to be a contraindication to taking HRT. Very few women with such conditions have taken HRT so research evidence is scarce. Women with such a history, but who require HRT should be referred to a specialist menopause clinic to discuss the treatment options. Occasionally HRT may be prescribed but under the close supervision of a specialist and only after a full discussion with the woman herself. Other treatments will also be discussed.

Undiagnosed abnormal vaginal bleeding

If a woman has experienced postmenopausal bleeding (i.e. bleeding more than 12 months after her last normal period) or if she has unexplained intermenstrual or post-coital bleeding, these should be investigated before HRT is commenced. In most instances investigation will not reveal any abnormal pathology and HRT can be commenced.

Liver disease

Severe, active liver disease is a contraindication to HRT (Whitehead and Godfree, 1992). If a woman has previously had mild liver disease it may be suggested that she has a non-oral type of HRT in order to avoid the 'first pass' effect on the liver.

PRINCIPLES OF HRT
– Contraindications

Pregnancy

Pregnancy can occur during the perimenopausal era and if the woman mistakes the resulting amenorrhoea as her menopause, HRT may be started inadvertently. If pregnancy is suspected, HRT should not be commenced.

Otosclerosis

This is a condition of progressive deafness which has been known to worsen during pregnancy and as no data are available regarding this condition and the use of HRT, caution is usually advised (Whitehead and Godfree, 1992).

Relative contraindications

Conditions which may need investigating prior to prescribing HRT are:

- Previous venous thrombosis
- Fibroids
- Endometriosis
- Untreated hypertension

Women with any of the above conditions can very often receive HRT but referral to a specialist centre may be necessary. Further investigations may need to be performed prior to HRT being prescribed.

Previous deep vein thrombosis (DVT)

Women who have experienced a DVT may receive HRT after a discussion of the known risks and benefits. Some studies have indicated that the risk of thrombosis may be increased in HRT users (Jick et al, 1996; Daly et al, 1996; Grodstein et al, 1996), although previous studies do not support this (Devor et al, 1992; Petitti et al, 1979; The Boston Collaborative Drug Surveillance Program, 1974). A clotting profile is performed and if abnormal, HRT withheld pending an expert haematological opinion. In the case of a recent DVT, specialist advice should be sought. Non-oral routes of HRT may be preferred. Further studies are needed to clarify the risk of thrombosis in HRT users, particularly those women with an existing thrombotic disorder.

Fibroids

After the menopause, fibroids usually shrink. The use of HRT may cause them to enlarge causing bleeding problems and discomfort. Ultrasound investigation will be helpful for monitoring fibroids whilst a woman is taking HRT. Small fibroids are not generally a problem.

Endometriosis

Endometriosis is a hormone-dependent disease. Even if it has previously been treated by surgery there is a small chance that HRT could cause it to recur. Careful monitoring is essential and women should be warned of the theoretical risk of the condition returning.

Untreated hypertension

Although HRT will not adversely effect blood pressure, it is generally advised that high blood pressure should be under control before HRT is commenced.

Other medical conditions

Gallstones

As the use of oestrogen can increase the risk of gallstones, women with gall bladder disease should be prescribed HRT with caution (Boston Collaborative Drug Surveillance Program, 1974).

Epilepsy

Some anti-epileptic drugs will enhance the metabolism of oral oestrogen. Higher doses or non-oral oestrogen may be necessary.

Previous myocardial infarct/angina

HRT does not appear to increase the risk of further cardiovascular incidents (Whitehead and Godfree, 1992).

Varicose veins

These are not worsened by HRT. Leg cramps are associated with HRT use, particularly in the early stages of treatment. Women themselves often perceive these as a problem and can be reassured.

Heavy smoker

Women should be encouraged to stop smoking for general health reasons, but a heavy smoker can still take HRT. Cardiovascular benefits would be even greater if she could also give up smoking. If a woman is experiencing profound menopausal symptoms, it may not be a diplomatic time to suggest that she should stop smoking!

Migraine

It is impossible to predict the affect of HRT on migraine. A trial of therapy may be necessary. Some women find that migraines improve after the menopause.

Diabetes

Diabetic women can safely take HRT, but glucose levels should be monitored in the early months of treatment in case adjustment of insulin is required. Theoretically, non-oral routes may be preferable.

THE BREAST ISSUE

Breast cancer is a common disease and appears to be hormone-related. Known risk factors for breast cancer are:

- Early menarche
- Late first pregnancy

- Late menopause
- Obesity (associated with higher levels of circulating oestrogen)

Anxiety about breast cancer and HRT is legitimate. Little agreement has been reached through clinical trials, although a large number of studies have been performed. Some studies have shown a slight increase in risk with HRT use (Colditz et al, 1990; Harris et al, 1992) whilst others have seen no change (Dupont and Page, 1991; Yang et al, 1992). General consensus is that there appears to be no risk with short-term use (up to 5 years) but there may be an increase in risk with HRT use of more than 10 years duration (Brinton et al, 1986; Steinberg et al, 1991; Colditz et al, 1995). The addition of a progestogen to oestrogen does not reduce the risk of breast cancer among postmenopausal women (Colditz et al, 1995).

If a woman develops breast cancer whilst she is taking HRT, her prognosis may be better than if she had not been taking the HRT (Bergkfist et al, 1989). Whether this is a true effect of HRT or whether it is due to the increased surveillance of women on HRT, is unclear. Neither is it of much consolation to a woman herself if she should develop a malignancy.

Family history of breast cancer

A woman with a strong family history of breast cancer is already at an increased risk herself. There is no evidence that such women increase their risk further if they take HRT, but few studies have been carried out on such women. These women are often prescribed HRT, after a full and frank discussion of the possible risks and with particular attention being paid to breast surveillance. For further information about breast monitoring see Chapter 7.

DURATION OF TREATMENT

How long a woman chooses to stay on HRT will largely depend on her reasons for taking it. Women with acute symptoms may only need HRT for a year or so before

PRINCIPLES OF HRT
— The breast issue
— Duration of treatment

Table 6.4   HRT products

Brand	Oestrogen	Progestogen	Type
Unopposed oestrogen			
Climaval	Oestradiol 1, 2 mg		Tablets
Estraderm	Oestradiol 25, 50, 100 μg		Patches
Estraderm MX	Oestradiol 25, 50, 75, 100 μg		Patches
Evorel	Oestradiol 25, 50, 100 μg		Patches
Fematrix	Oestradiol 40, 80 μg		Patches
Femseven	Oestradiol 50 μg		Patches
Harmogen	Oestrone 0.93 mg		Tablets
Hormonin	Oestradiol/oestriol/oestrone		Tablets
Menorest	Oestradiol 37.5, 50, 75 μg		Patches
Oestrogel	Oestradiol 1.5 mg		Gel
Premarin	Conjugated oestrogen 0.625, 1.25 mg		Tablets
Progynova	Oestradiol 1, 2 mg		Tablets
Progynova TS	Oestradiol 50, 100 μg		Patches
Zumenon	Oestradiol 2 mg		Tablets
Implants	Oestradiol 25, 50, 100 mg		Implants
Gonadomimetic			
Livial	Tibolone 2.5 mg		Tablets
Sequential combined			
Climagest	Oestradiol 1, 2 mg	Norethisterone 1 mg	Tablets
Cycloprogynova	Oestradiol 1, 2 mg	Levonorgestrel 0.25, 0.5 mg	Tablets

Estracombi	Oestradiol 50 µg	Norethisterone 250 µg	Patches
Estrapak	Oestradiol 50 µg	Norethisterone 1 mg	Patches/tablets
Evorel-Pak	Oestradiol 50 µg	Norethisterone 1 mg	Patches/tablets
Femapak	Oestradiol 80 µg	Dydrogesterone 10 mg	Patches/tablets
Femosten	Oestradiol 1, 2 mg	Dydrogesterone 10, 20 mg	Tablets
Improvera	Oestrone 0.93 mg	Medroxyprogesterone 10 mg	Tablets
Menophase	Mestranol	Norethisterone 1 mg	Tablets
Nuvelle	Oestradiol 2 mg	Levonorgestrel 75 µg	Tablets
Premique Cycle	Conjugated oestrogens 0.625 mg	Medroxyprogesterone 10 mg	Tablets
Trisequens	Oestradiol/oestriol 2, 4 mg	Norethisterone 1 mg	Tablets
Tridestra	Oestradiol 2 mg	Medoxyprogesterone 20 mg (trycyclical)	Tablets

Continuous combined

Kliofem	Oestradiol 2 mg	Norethisterone 1 mg	Tablets
Premique	Conjugated oestrogens 0.625 mg	Medroxyprogesterone 5 mg	Tablets
Climesse	Oestradiol 2 mg	Norethisterone 0.7 mg	Tablets

Local treatments

Estring	Oestradiol		Vaginal ring
Ortho Dienoestrol	Dienoestrol		Vaginal cream
Ortho Gynest	Oestriol		Vaginal cream pessary
Ovestin	Oestriol		Vaginal cream
Premarin	Conjugated oestrogen		Vaginal cream
Vagifem	Oestradiol		Vaginal tablets

symptoms resolve. Others may stop HRT after 2 years only to find that menopausal symptoms return because they are still in the climacteric. For long-term protection of heart and bone, treatment is recommended for at least 5 years. Women wanting to stay on HRT for more than 10 years need an open discussion with regard to risks and benefits, particularly in relation to breast cancer. Currently, many women take HRT for only a few months because of unacceptable side-effects. Although this is a personal decision, you should encourage women to return for a consultation prior to stopping HRT. A change in regimen may be all that is needed.

How to stop

Women wanting to stop HRT may fear that their symptoms will suddenly return. If HRT is stopped suddenly, some women will experience symptoms as a result of the rapidly falling oestrogen levels. For this reason it is often suggested that the oestrogen be tailed off gradually over a period of a few weeks. Initially the dose can be reduced, then tablets can be taken on alternate days or patches changed less frequently. Meanwhile the progestogen is continued as normal. Once all oestrogen has been stopped, the progestogen can be discontinued at the end of a course. Women discontinuing HRT after oestrogen implants should be advised to continue progestogen until withdrawal bleeding ceases.

REFERENCES

Archer DF, Pickar JH, Bottiglioni F et al (1994) Bleeding patterns in postmenopausal women taking continuous combined or sequential regimens of conjugated estrogens with medoxyprogesterone acetate. *Obstet. Gynaecol.* 83:5(1) 686–692.

Benedek-Jaszmann LJ (1987) Long term placebo controlled efficacy and safety study of ORG OD 14 in climacteric women. *Maturitas* (suppl. 1): 25–33.

Bergkfist L, Adami HO, Persson I et al (1989) The risk of breast cancer in postmenopausal women who have used estrogen replacement therapy. *J. Am. Med. Assoc.* 321: 293–297.

Boston Collaborative Drug Surveillance Program (1974) Surgically confirmed cases of gall bladder disease, venous thromboembolism and breast tumours in relation to postmenopausal estrogen therapy. *N Engl. J. Med.* **290**: 15–18.

Brinton LA, Hoover RN & Fraumeni JF (1986) Menopausal oestrogens and breast cancer risk: An expanded case-control study. *Br. J. Cancer* **54**: 825–832.

Colditz GA et al (1990) Prospective study of estrogen replacement therapy and risk of breast cancer in postmenopausal women. *J. Am. Med. Assoc.* **264**: 2648–2653.

Colditz GA, Hankinson SE, Hunter DJ et al (1995) The use of oestrogen and progestins and the risk of breast cancer in postmenopausal women. *N Engl. J. Med.* **332**: 1589–1593.

Daly E, Vessey MP, Hawkins MM et al (1996) Risk of venous thromboembolism in users of hormone replacement therapy. *Lancet* **348**: 977–980.

Devor M, Barrett-Connor E, Renvall M, Feigal Jr D & Ramsdell J (1992) Estrogen replacement therapy and the risk of venous thrombosis. *Am. J. Med.* **92**: 275–282.

Dupont WD & Page DL (1991) Menopausal estrogen replacement therapy and breast cancer. *Arch. Int. Med.* **151**: 67–72.

Ettinger B, Selby J & Citron JT (1994) Cyclic HRT using quarterly progestin. *Obstet. Gynaecol.* **83**: 693–700.

Gangar K, Cust M & Whitehead MI (1989) Symptoms of oestrogen deficiency with supraphysiological levels of plasma oestradiol concentrations in women with oestradiol implants. *Br. Med. J.* **299**: 601.

Grodstein F, Stampfer MJ, Goldhaber SZ et al (1996) Prospective study of exogenous hormones and risk of pulmonary embolism. *Lancet* **348**: 983–987.

Harris RE, Namboodiri KK & Wynder EL (1992) Breast cancer risk: Effects of estrogen replacement therapy and body mass. *J. Natl. Cancer Inst.* **84**: 1575–1582.

Henderson BE (1989) The Cancer Question: An overview of recent epidemiological and retrospective data. *Am. J. Obstet. Gynecol.* **161**: 1859.

Hirvonen E, Salmi T, Puolakka J et al (1995) Can progestin be limited to every third month only in postmenopausal women taking estrogen? *Maturitas* **21**: 39–44.

Jick H, Derby L, Myers MW et al (1996) Risk of hospital admission for ideopathic venous thromboembolism among users of postmenopausal oestrogens. *Lancet* **348**: 981–983.

Lievertz RW (1987) Pharmacology and pharmokinetics of oestrogens. *Am. J. Obstet. Gynecol.* **156**: 1289–1293.

Magos AL, Brincat M, Studd JWW et al (1985) Amenorrhoea and endometrial atrophy with continuous oral oestrogen and progestogen therapy in postmenopausal women. *Obstet. Gynecol.* **65**: 496–499.

Mashchak CA, Lobo RA, Dozono-Takano R et al (1982) Comparison of pharmacodynamic properties of various oestrogen formulations. *Am. J. Obstet. Gynecol.* **144**: 511–518.

Persson I, Adani HO, Bergkfist L et al (1989) Risk of endometrial cancer after treatment with oestrogens alone or in conjunction with progestogens: Results of a prospective study. *Br. Med. J.* **298**: 147–151.

Petitti DB, Wingerd J, Pellegrin F & Ramcharan S (1979) Risk of vascular disease in women: smoking, oral contraceptives, noncontraceptives estrogens and other factors. *JAMA* **242**: 1150–1154.

Rymer J (1992) Tibolone: Alternative relief for postmenopausal symptoms. *J. Sex. Health* **2**(5): 25–27.

Siddle NC (1989) Psychological effects of different progestogens. In *Concensus Development Conference on Progestogens, International Proceedings Journal* **1**: 214–217.

Silverberg SG (1988) Hyperplasia and carcinome of the endometrium. *Semin. Diagnostic Pathol.* **5**: 135–153.

Stern MD (1982) Pharmacology of conjugated oestrogens. *Maturitas* **4**: 333–339.

Steinberg KK, Thacker SB, Smith SJ et al. (1991) A meta analysis of the effects of estrogen replacement therapy on the risk of breast cancer. *J. Am. Med. Assoc.* **265**: 1985.

Sturdee DW, Wade-Evans T, Paterson MEL et al (1978) Relations between bleeding pattern, endometrial histology and oestrogen treatment in postmenopausal women. *Br. Med. J.* 1 1575–1577.

Upton V (1988) Contraception in the woman over 40. In Studd JWW & Whitehead MI (eds) *The Menopause*, pp. 289–304. Oxford: Blackwell Scientific Publications.

Whitehead MI, Hillard TC & Crook D (1990) The role and use of progestogens. *Obstet. Gynecol.* **75**: 595–765.

Whitehead MI & Godfree V (1992) *Hormone Replacement Therapy – Your Questions Answered.* London: Churchill Livingstone.

Whitehead MI, Whitcroft SJ & Hillard TC (1993) Atlas of the menopause (Encyclopaedia of Visual Medicine Series) 25.

Yang CT et al (1992) Non contraceptive hormone use and risk of breast cancer. *Cancer, Causes and Control* **3**: 475–479.

Chapter 7

Practical Aspects of Hormone Replacement Therapy

Ten years ago, the prescribing of hormone replacement therapy and discussion of menopause issues was confined mainly to consultations with general practitioners or occasional visits to gynaecology departments. Women experiencing severe menopausal symptoms might have received HRT, but other women simply 'put up with the symptoms'. If a woman sought the help of her doctor, she was fortunate if she got more than a 10 minute consultation and a prescription.

Fortunately, times have changed in all areas of medicine and perhaps women's health is one area which has seen more changes than any other. Women themselves are demanding an improved service from healthcare professionals, particularly when it comes to issues such as the menopause. The choice of whether to take HRT has, to a large extent, been removed from the prescriber to the individual woman, who now makes the choice herself after consideration of all the necessary information and facts. The doctor still has the final say after assessing the woman but the decision is more likely to have been made jointly, after greater discussion between doctor and patient. The nurse, particularly the practice nurse, sits conveniently between patient and doctor. She is often the facilitator in the decision-making process. The woman will not take HRT until she has all the information she needs and the doctor will not prescribe it unless he/she is confident that it is safe and appropriate. The nurse can be involved both in helping the woman to make an informed choice and in ensuring that the necessary procedures are carried out before treatment starts. Broadly speaking the nurse's role falls into three categories:

- Informing women about the menopause and HRT
- Preparing a woman to take HRT
- Monitoring and assessing the woman who is taking HRT

INFORMING WOMEN

Before a woman can make what is described as an 'informed choice', she needs the necessary information to help her make the decision wisely. Many women discover that gathering accurate information about the menopause and HRT is a difficult task. They often have to choose between a medical textbook, which is dauntingly detailed, or a magazine article which emphasizes either the horrors or the miracles of HRT. Balanced articles and books are hard to find if you are not sure where to start looking. Increasingly the nurse in general practice is becoming the person women will turn to for unbiased but accurate knowledge. It is therefore vital that nurses are well informed about the risks and benefits of HRT and that they keep up to date with current research. The subject of menopause and HRT is a vast one, so what do you choose to tell women and how do you impart the information? How do you ensure that the women who really need the information receive it, and how do you reach across barriers of class, education and race so that all women have the necessary information for themselves?

Issues to cover when considering what women need to know in order to make an informed choice about HRT are:

- Understanding of the menopause
- Dispelling myths
- Unrealistic expectations
- Understanding HRT
- Anticipating anxieties

Understanding the menopause

It is sometimes necessary to spend time explaining a little about the female reproductive system so that each woman has a better understanding about what is happening to her body. For some women this will enable them to have a better understanding of HRT and how it is used to replace the oestrogen which their own body is no longer producing. Women who have little understanding of how their body works may be more likely to have concerns about the effects of HRT.

Dispelling myths

There are many old wives' tales about the menopause and many beliefs about HRT which are widely held but inaccurate. These need to be discussed and corrected. Some of the myths relate to a misunderstanding about what HRT actually does, whilst the old wives' tales may be passed from mother to daughter or friend to friend. Repeated often enough they begin to sound like authoritative statements and can be difficult to dispel.

If you started your periods late, you will get a bad (or good) menopause.
Age of menarche has no influence on subsequent menopausal symptoms.

If your mother had a bad menopause, then you will too.

This is not necessarily true, although a particularly early or late menopause may run in families.

If you live a healthy lifestyle, you can avoid unpleasant menopause symptoms.

If only this were true! Menopausal symptoms may affect the fittest and healthiest women as well as the 'couch potatoes'. A healthy lifestyle is always to be commended but will not guarantee you a trouble-free menopause.

If you could not take the contraceptive pill, then you cannot take HRT.

This is a widely held belief which has arisen from a basic misunderstanding about how HRT differs from the contraceptive pill.

If you have never been pregnant you will delay your menopause.

This is untrue; parity is unrelated to time of menopause.

If you take HRT, you will simply make things worse when you stop.

HRT does not postpone symptoms, but overrides them, so providing treatment is taken for long enough, symptoms should not be worse when HRT is stopped.

These and other myths about menopause and HRT are commonplace and it can be a hard job convincing women that what they have heard is wrong and that what you are telling them is right! This is one reason to provide good quality literature about the subject so that women can take it away, read it and return with the questions.

Unrealistic expectations

The glamour issue

Some women start HRT with false expectations of what it will do for them. They may have read media reports of how HRT will keep them young and be hoping that the wrinkles and greying hairs will disappear. If so, they are certain to be disappointed when they discover that, even after taking HRT, they do not look 10 years younger! However HRT may have a positive effect on sleep pattern, perhaps making the woman look and feel less tired and giving her more energy to live her life. It is helpful to have discussed this issue, particularly with women who seem to be asking for HRT primarily for this reason.

Which symptoms will be improved?

There are some symptoms which are very common at the time of the menopause and which respond very well to HRT in nearly all women, e.g. hot flushes and night sweats. There are other symptoms which can arise at this time which may or may not respond to HRT, depending on the underlying cause. An example would be poor memory: some women find that this improves with HRT, others do not and it would be wrong to mislead women into thinking that all loss of memory will improve once HRT is started. It is well worth taking the time to help the woman consider her symptoms and try to assess which are likely to improve with HRT and which are not. No promises can be made, but after discussion it some- times transpires that certain symptoms have not actually arisen at this time, but have always been a problem. In this case it is unlikely that HRT will help.

Hot flushes are usually the first symptoms to improve with HRT use, other symptoms may take much longer and women should be warned that their symptoms will not disappear overnight but that some symptoms may take weeks or even months to improve.

Understanding HRT

The word 'hormone' can be off-putting to some women as they associate it with harmful and unwanted effects. Women who are familiar with the contraceptive pill may confuse it with hormone replacement therapy and draw the wrong conclusions about HRT. The woman who is told at age 35 years to stop the contraceptive pill because she is a smoker will be confused when at the age of 50 years she is advised to consider HRT in order to prevent heart disease. A simple explanation about the difference between 'synthetic' and 'natural' HRT is required.

Most women will understand that HRT consists of oestrogen, but some may not realize that progestogen is also often given. It is important that the woman who has not had a hysterectomy understands the need for a progestogen alongside the oestrogen. Women should be warned of the possible effects of the progestogen and in particular the likely timing of the withdrawal bleed, if appropriate. Once it has been decided which HRT a woman will take, it is helpful to explain to her which part of the treatment is oestrogen and which is progestogen. This will enable her to clearly identify the components of her own treatment and so be able to relate the side-effects to one or the other component. It also means that with some therapies she will be able occasionally to alter the timing of her bleed if it is inconvenient. Most HRT preparations are packaged in a 'user friendly' way, but women may still need an explanation of how to take the treatment. This i especially so for the non-oral preparations which are a less familiar way of taking medication for most women.

Many women do not realize that HRT is not simply one medication but a variety of doses, types and regimens. It is important that you stress to women that the first preparation they try may not be the one which is most suited to them and that some adjustment or 'tailoring' of the dose may be necessary.

Concern about side-effects is the commonest reason given for stopping HRT (NOP, 1991). Yet in many instances, it is not the actual side-effects which are unbearable (although this is occasionally the case), but rather the underlying anxieties caused by the side-effects which make a woman consider stopping her HRT. For example, the woman with breast tenderness fears that she may be getting breast cancer, the women with leg cramps fears she is developing a thrombosis and a woman with headaches is frightened of having a stroke.

Side-effects in the early weeks of starting any form of HRT are common and you should prepare women to experience them. They usually subside on their own, but occasionally a change in dose or type of HRT is required. Women who are prepared for these early side-effects are more likely to stay on the treatment if they understand that they are common and not dangerous. With as many as two-thirds of women stopping HRT in the first 6 months (Hall and Spector, 1992), primarily because of side-effects, it is particularly important that those women who are recommended HRT for osteoporosis or cardiovascular protection realize that short-term HRT is unlikely to confer much benefit. These women especially should be encouraged to return to the clinic if they have problems, rather than simply stopping treatment.

Anticipating anxieties

When a woman comes to discuss the issue of HRT it is likely that she will have lots of questions to ask and perhaps some concerns to express. Some women will have anxieties in their minds which they are hesitant to raise, either because they do not want to look foolish or simply because they are hoping that you will raise it first. It is therefore helpful to address commonly-held anxieties with all women as well as encouraging women to ask specifically about those issues which are of concern to them individually. Such issues include:

Fear of cancer

The issue of cancer, and in particular breast cancer is very important to all women. Most women would not take HRT if it was shown that any use at all caused an increase risk of breast cancer. This fear is not helped by many media articles which have exacerbated fears by printing 'scare stories' which are biased or unproven. Even if the matter is not raised by a woman herself, it is a good subject to discuss as it gives the opportunity for education about 'breast awareness' and stressing the need for mammography in women over 50 years old. It is reassuring to be able to remind women that a balanced form of HRT, containing oestrogen and progestogen will prevent a build up of the womb lining and so reduce risk of endometrial cancer. You can also advise her that the risk of female cancers such as ovary, cervix and fallopian tubes are is not increased with the use of HRT. For information on HRT and the risk of breast cancer, see Chapter 6.

Weight gain

Many women fear that by starting HRT they will suddenly have a dramatic uncontrollable rise in weight. For the woman already facing a struggle with her weight the prospect of gaining more can be quite alarming. There is certainly no evidence that HRT causes a significant weight gain in most women taking it (Nachtigall et al, 1979). Some women do gain weight after starting HRT but it is impossible to know whether the HRT itself was the cause.

Risk of thrombosis

Fear of thrombosis whilst taking HRT has arisen because of the confusion which many women have about the difference between the contraceptive pill and HRT. Some women may have been advised in the past that they should not take HRT, when in fact it would be quite safe for them to do so. These women will need careful counselling and perhaps referral to a specialist in order to be sure that the treatment they are being offered is safe for them to take.

Bleeding

The return of a monthly bleed is a major drawback with many types of HRT. You should warn women when to expect their bleed, reassuring them that it should not be too heavy or painful and that if the regimen is carefully balanced, the bleed will be easily predicted each month. If a woman is truly postmenopausal (as opposed to perimenopausal), you should discuss the option of a 'no-bleed' treatment (see Chapter 6).

Fertility

You should remind women that HRT will not act as a contraceptive and the perimenopausal woman will need to

Table 7.1   Investigations prior to starting HRT

Medical history
Symptom history
Height/weight
Blood pressure
Breast examination
Pelvic examination

continue using a contraceptive method whilst taking HRT (see Chapter 5). However, you can also reassure the postmenopausal woman that the return of a monthly bleed does not indicate the return of fertility.

INFORMATION – HOW WILL YOU GIVE IT?

Once you have decided that you want to improve awareness among all women approaching the menopause with whom you have contact, you are faced with trying to decide the best way of doing it. There is in fact no 'best' way and you may need to experiment to see what works best for you and your patients. Many ways have been tried and what is successful in one area of practice may not work well somewhere else. Here are a few ideas which other nurses have used, you may like to try them yourself or perhaps adapt them to your own situation.

Ideas for providing information

- Group sessions (open or by invitation)
- Individual targeting of women (by age or risk assessment)
- Loan of books and videos
- Free literature
- Dedicated clinic session (open or by invitation)
- Opportunistic moments

These are discussed more fully in Chapter 9.

PREPARING A WOMAN TO TAKE HRT

Any woman who has made the decision to consider HRT, ideally after being fully informed, wants to be sure that the treatment will be safe for her to take and that she will be adequately monitored whilst on therapy. Certain tests are routinely carried out prior to HRT being prescribed and whilst the woman is taking it. It often falls to the nurse to carry out these tests and to answer questions arising from them.

Investigations prior to HRT

Medical history

In general practice, a full medical history will already be available in the patients records, but at other clinics it will be necessary to ask the patient directly about issues which might contraindicate the use of HRT. It may also reveal other reasons why HRT should be considered, e.g. family history of heart disease or osteoporosis. After taking a full history the nurse or doctor may decide that further investigations are required before HRT is started.

Symptom history

If a woman is presenting with climacteric symptoms, it may seem obvious to give the woman time to describe them. However women themselves have complained that they often have little opportunity to talk about what they are experiencing. A 'listening ear' can be therapeutic in itself and for some women, the reassurance that what they are experiencing is common, is enough to alleviate anxiety. Taking a good history before treatment also helps to evaluate the effectiveness of a treatment at a later date. Symptom charts and questionnaires can be helpful in some circumstances.

Height/weight

A baseline height measurement will be useful if a woman is at high risk of osteoporosis for monitoring purposes. Measuring weight as well enables you to calculate body mass index, which is useful for purposes of general health advice. If a woman is very overweight or underweight you may decide to offer specific help with this issue, but it is unlikely to influence the prescribing of HRT. Another reason to measure a woman's weight is so that there is a record of her pretreatment weight if she thinks the HRT is causing her to gain weight.

Blood pressure

Uncontrolled hypertension should be detected and treated before HRT is started. Very rarely HRT causes a rapid rise in blood pressure in the first few weeks of treatment, so a baseline measurement is essential (Whitehead and Godfree, 1992).

Breast examination

Breast examination is often performed by the prescribing doctor in order to rule out any pre-existing lumps or abnormalities, which would need investigating before HRT was started. Mammography is not routinely recommended before starting HRT, except for women considered to be at a high risk for breast cancer. All women over 50 years should be encouraged to have 3-yearly mammograms as recommended by the guidelines of the National Breast Screening programme, whether or not they are taking HRT.

Pelvic examination

Bimanual pelvic examination should be performed prior to starting HRT to rule out obvious pelvic pathology, such as ovarian cysts or fibroids. If any abnormality is found, it should be investigated before HRT is started. Additional cervical smears are unnecessary unless clinically indicated.

PRACTICAL ASPECTS OF HRT — Preparing a woman

Summary of extra investigations that may be required

- Thyroid function test
- Clotting screen
- Lipid profile
- Mammography
- Follicle stimulating hormone level
- Bone densitometry
- Endometrial assessment

Thyroid function test (TFT)

Symptoms of thyroid deficiency may be similar to climacteric symptoms and often affect women in mid life, so occasionally a TFT is performed to make a differential diagnosis.

Clotting screen

This is important for those women who have had a previous thrombosis, or who have a strong family history of thrombosis.

Lipid profile

This is useful in women who have a strong family history of heart disease. The results may give an indication *for* HRT rather than against it.

Mammography

All women over 50 years are encouraged to be part of the National Breast Screening programme, but some women may need a pretreatment mammogram or referral to a specialist before starting HRT. Such women would be those with a strong family history of breast cancer (i.e. a first degree relative) or women who already have some evidence of breast disease.

Table 7.2   Ongoing assessments for women on HRT

Weight
Blood pressure
Symptom assessment
Side-effect assessment
Monitoring of bleeding
Breast examination if appropriate
Pelvic examination if appropriate
Question time

Follicle stimulating hormone level

These measurements are useful in the hysterectomized woman who is experiencing less typical climacteric symptoms and are important in the diagnosis of premature menopause. Single levels are unlikely to be reliable, so serial measurements should be performed.

Bone densitometry

This test is not available to all National Health patients. If available it is useful for those women who may be at risk of osteoporosis but will only take HRT if that risk could be demonstrated.

Endometrial assessment

If a woman has experienced abnormal bleeding, such as heavy, prolonged periods or if she has experienced a post-menopausal bleed (i.e. 12 months or more since her last period), assessment of the endometrium may be required. An endometrial sample may be taken or ultrasound used to measure the endometrial thickness.

In most instances the primary healthcare team will carry out the relevant tests, but there will be some women who will need referral to a specialist menopause clinic. These might include:

- Women with previous breast cancer or a first degree relative with the disease

HRT 'does not make women fat'

BY JEREMY LAURANCE

LONG-TERM use of hormone replacement therapy to counter the effects of the menopause does not lead to an increase in weight, researchers have found.

Fear of weight gain is one of the principal reasons why women refuse HRT or give it up soon after starting. However, the first study to examine the long-term effects of the treatment has found no evidence that it adds pounds.

One in five post-menopausal women in Britain is given HRT and the proportion is expected to grow to one in three by the end of the decade. But there is a widespread belief among women and doctors that the reduction in menopausal symptoms is bought at the expense of an increase in girth.

Researchers from the University of California studied 671 women over almost 20 years to 1991. Their results, published in *The Journal of the American Medical Association*, showed that there were no differences between users and non-users of HRT on measures of obesity, fat distribution or body composition.

Figure 7.1   Many women are concerned about weight gain on HRT. (*The Times*, 3rd Jan. 1996.)

- Women with a history of several thromboses
- Women with a complicated medical history
- Women with a premature menopause
- Women with concurrent gynaecological problems, such as fibroids, endometriosis or abnormal bleeding
- Women who have already tried many types of HRT with little success

MONITORING AND EVALUATION OF HRT

Initial evaluation should be offered to women after about 3–4 months on therapy, or after changing to a new regimen. By this time, early side-effects should have subsided and a regular pattern of bleeding should be established with a cyclical regimen. If side-effects have persisted after this time, it may be necessary to consider a change of regimen.

Once a woman is established on a satisfactory treatment, with few side-effects and an acceptable bleed, if appropriate, follow up visits can be reduced to twice a year, or sooner if problems arise.

Ongoing assessments

Weight

For some women, the prospect of gaining weight whilst taking HRT is a real anxiety. Being weighed on the same (hopefully accurate!) scales can be reassuring. For women who have a long-standing weight problem, it can be an ordeal to be weighed at each visit and is probably unnecessary in many instances. Being overweight will not, in itself, be a reason to tell a woman to stop her HRT. Measurement of weight is performed as a general health check rather than because the decision to continue HRT rests on the outcome, so you need to be sensitive to all women and think before you routinely weigh all women at every visit. If a woman does gain weight whilst taking HRT, it is worth trying to establish whether it is cyclical (i.e. progestogen related), in which case that component of the therapy can be changed. Some apparent bloatedness can occur with the use of HRT but this is most likely to be demonstrated by a tightening of rings or the waistband rather than a noticeable weight gain. A change of treatment may resolve this. For some women, the feeling of weight gain may be a reflection of fuller breasts and a return to a more normal female fat distribution, i.e. around the hips and thighs rather than the abdomen.

Blood pressure

It has become established practice to record the blood pressure of women who take HRT, yet there is no good evidence that it will be altered simply by the use of HRT

(Utian, 1978; Wren and Routledge, 1983). Women who gain weight may see a rise in blood pressure. If hypertension is detected whilst a woman is taking HRT, she will need assessment and treatment for her blood pressure in its own right.

Symptom assessment

It is helpful for a woman to review her symptoms once she is settled on HRT. Some symptoms may have disappeared, others may be improving and yet others may not have been affected at all. A symptom assessment scale can help a woman to recognize those symptoms which may have decreased in intensity, even those symptoms which may have decreased in intensity, even though they have not disappeared altogether. A chart will also help you to raise those symptoms which the woman may be embarrassed to discuss, yet which could be troublesome, for instance, bladder symptoms or sexual concerns. It can also be reassuring for a woman to be able to look back at a previous chart and recognize how much she has improved, perhaps without even realizing at the time. Occasionally an increase in dose will be necessary in order to further improve general symptoms.

Side-effects

If a woman has received adequate information before starting HRT, she will hopefully have reached her initial assessment visit without stopping treatment. By this time, side-effects should be diminishing and a more accurate assessment of the suitability of her HRT will be possible. If she is still experiencing side-effects, a change of HRT may be required.

It is important to try and establish, by direct questioning, when side-effects occur. Oestrogen-related side-effects are often continuous and can be relieved by adjusting the dose or changing the type or route of oestrogen. Progestogenic effects often persist for as long as that particular progestogen is taken, again a change in dose or type of progestogen may be needed. There are established doses of progestogen which are considered to offer endometrial protection and few doctors will recommend a lower dose than this, except in unusual circumstances. The duration of cyclical progestogen is also unlikely to be altered except by a specialist, but sometimes changing to a different progestogen is sufficient to reduce unwanted effects.

In cases of severe progestogenic side-effects and under the guidance of a specialist, it may be suggested that more radical steps be taken, such as prescribing oestrogen alone, or even offering a hysterectomy. These are controversial issues and decisions which are likely to be made by a specialist who can offer the necessary support and follow-up which may be necessary.

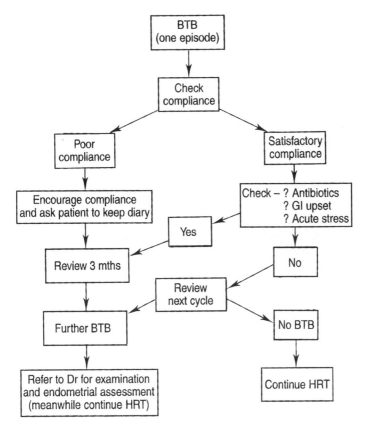

Figure 7.2   Guidelines for the management of breakthrough bleeding on cyclical HRT.

Table 7.3   Indications for extra pelvic examination

Postcoital bleeding
Irregular bleeding
Pelvic pain
Episodes of intermenstrual bleeding

Some women experience so-called side-effects which are minor but troublesome. These can often be resolved if the woman is given opportunity to express them. Usually they relate to the practicalities of taking the medication and are common in women using patches or creams. Patches which persistently fall off or cause a minor irritation can be a result of a woman not using them correctly. For instance, she may be applying the patch to wet skin, or over talcum powder not realizing that this will affect how well they stick. A nurse who is working with women using HRT will soon pick up a host of 'tips', which whilst unscientific in origin, can be passed on to women in the hope that sometimes it may make the taking of HRT less troublesome.

Withdrawal bleed

At each follow-up visit, a woman taking a cyclical regimen of HRT should be directly asked about her withdrawal bleed. It is important because if the bleed is abnormal, it could be a sign that the dose of HRT needs adjusting. It is also good to find out whether the bleed is what you would normally expect with use of HRT and whether it is acceptable to the woman herself. You should discuss the following issues:

Timing. Does the bleed occur at the time you would expect it for the regimen she is taking? It is normal for the bleed to start at, or near, the end of the course of progestogen or a couple of days later. A very early or late onset of a bleed may indicate the need for a change in therapy (Whitehead and Hillard Crook, 1990).

Intensity. The bleed should not be unacceptably heavy and is normally similar to or lighter than a normal period. Some women will only experience a very light bleed or even no bleeding at all. This is considered normal, although some specialists would recommend that an ultrasound be performed, showing endometrial thickness. An over-thickened endometrium would indicate the need for further investigation to ensure that safety of the endometrium is being maintained. A change of progestogen may be necessary. You should also check that the regimen is being correctly taken and that the progestogen is not being missed either through error or intentionally.

Duration. Withdrawal bleeds commonly last up to 7 days, with many women experiencing bleeding for only 2 or 3 days, once they are established on treatment.

Irregular bleeding. You should ask whether any extra bleeding has occurred outside the normal monthly bleed. Mid-cycle bleeding on a regular basis, or postcoital bleeding should be investigated. Occasional irregular bleeding could be caused by concurrent medications such as antibiotics, or by a stomach upset causing a disturbance in absorption. Even stress may cause a one-off episode of irregular bleeding. If you consider that the bleed is not as it should be, the woman will need to see the doctor with a view to a change of treatment or further investigation.

Breast examination

In most menopause clinics it is normal practice to perform a breast check on women who are taking HRT, usually on an annual basis. There has been no research to show that this is of particular benefit to women on HRT, other than to reassure both doctor and patient that no obvious lumps are present. However, it would seem a reasonable procedure, considering that it is painless, minimally invasive and quick. Many women find it reassuring to have a breast check from a 'professional' even if they themselves are 'breast aware'. If you find a lump, the woman would be referred for urgent breast assessment. It should be stressed that an annual check by a nurse or doctor cannot replace the need for every woman to be aware of changes in her own breasts. Nurses may take this opportunity to encourage 'breast awareness'.

Pelvic examination

There is no need for extra routine pelvic examinations just because a woman is taking HRT. Some specialists ensure that one is performed three yearly along with cervical cytology. Occasionally there will be a clinical indication for an extra examination and you may need to refer the woman to the doctor in these instances.

Question time

When a woman returns to clinic for a routine follow up, there is a tendency to carry out the necessary procedures, ask the relevant questions and move on to the next patient. HRT is a medication which is not usually being taken for a life-threatening disease and monitoring a

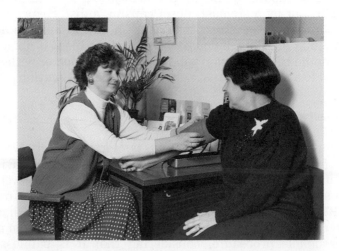

Figure 7.3   Woman being assessed. (Courtesy of the Medical Illustration Department, Northwick Park Institute for Medical Research, Northwick Park Hospital, Harrow, Middlesex.)

woman on therapy can appear very routine. Women may have questions which they want to ask, but often feel that the opportunity to do so does not present itself. Women may wish to discuss whether to come off treatment or may have minor anxieties which could be easily allayed. It is therefore helpful to make a point of asking each woman whether there are any issues she would like to discuss. Opportunity is then given for women to ask those questions which, in themselves are probably not medically important, but which once answered, enable the woman to feel more confident about her treatment. Such issues may include:

• Media coverage of HRT
• Underlying anxieties about breast cancer
• Advice received from 'friends'
• Practical issues about taking her HRT

Nurse or doctor?

In the past, women on HRT expected to see a doctor regularly for monitoring and assessment. Now that practice nurses are becoming much more involved in the care and assessment of all patients, it is common for them to be doing some of the monitoring of treatment. In the same way that nurses trained in Family Planning will care for women on the contraceptive pill, suitably trained nurses could do much of the routine monitoring of HRT. As well as releasing the time for their doctor colleagues, it will more importantly lead to a 'team approach' in caring for women at the time of the menopause. Many women will be pleased to have the opportunity to see the nurse rather than the doctor on some occasions, particularly as it is not uncommon for them to have longer (more realistic) appointment times, which are more conducive to discussion (Quantock and Beynon, 1995).

As with all areas of medicine, it is important that the nurse recognizes her own limitations and establishes guidelines as to when referral back to a doctor is necessary. It is useful to have a protocol agreed by doctors and nurses within a team, so that all staff involved are

PRACTICAL ASPECTS OF HRT
– Monitoring & evaluation

working to agreed and consistent standards of care (see Chapter 9).

When to refer to a doctor

- Poorly controlled symptoms
- Unmanageable or unexpected side-effects
- On discovery of a breast lump
- Abnormal bleeding pattern
- At a woman's own request

Alternate visits

It has become practice in some clinics for a woman on HRT to alternate between the doctor or practice nurse for follow-up visits. In this instance, she would then see the doctor on an annual basis, with a visit to the nurse in between. Many women express satisfaction at this system, as they feel confident that any problems will be detected yet feel that they do not actually need to see the doctor every time. Some women find nurses more approachable about minor issues which they may not feel able to discuss with their doctors. Women are very aware of the pressured appointment times and may take the opportunity to discuss issues with the nurse that they have not discussed with the doctor. Some women feel intimidated by the medical profession and yet will open up a discussion with a nurse, perhaps because they feel more on the 'same wavelength'.

There will always be those few women who feel 'short-changed' if they do not see a doctor at each visit, however well qualified and experienced the nurse may be. It can be difficult to persuade such women to see a nurse at any visit. You will work out your own way of dealing with such women; I simply pass them on to the doctor and let them get on with it!

The assessment of a woman prior to starting HRT and the ongoing monitoring thereafter is a satisfying part of the nurse's work. Many women will present with a number of problems, sometimes unable to clarify for themselves which are hormone-related and which are not. Spending time with such women is time well spent and women themselves are often very grateful for the help and advice they get. Time spent advising a woman before she starts treatment may save time later and also ensures that the woman is in a position to make a truly informed choice about HRT. Preparing women fully for HRT will result in women who have realistic expectations and subsequently are less likely to simply stop treatment after only a short while. This is particularly relevant to those women considering long-term HRT.

REFERENCES

Hall G & Spector TD (1992) Hormone Replacement Therapy – Why do so few women use it. *Osteoporosis Review* **1**: 2.

National Opinion Poll Survey (1991) *The Menopause Revolution, how far have we come?*

Nachtigall LE, Nachtigall RH & Nachtigall RB (1979) Estrogen replacement therapy II – A prospective study in the relationship to carcinoma and metabolic problems. *Obstet. Gynecol.* **54**: 74–79.

Quantock C & Beynon J (1995) HRT and the nurse counsellor. *Nursing Standard* **9**:(40), 20–21.

Utian W (1978) Effect of postmenopausal oestrogen therapy on diastolic blood pressure and body weight. *Maturitas* **1**: 3.

Whitehead MI & Godfree V (1992) *HRT – Your Questions Answered.* London: Churchill Livingstone.

Whitehead MI & Hillard Crook D (1990) The role and use of progestogens. *Obstet. Gynecol.* **75**(suppl. 4): 59s–79s.

Wren BG & Routledge AD (1983) The effect of type and dose of oestrogen on the blood pressure of postmenopausal women. *Maturitas* **5**: 135–142.

Chapter 8

Nonhormonal Management of the Menopause

HRT successfully alleviates menopausal symptoms, both physical and psychological (Coope et al, 1975; Dennerstein, 1988; Hunt, 1988) as well as conferring long-term benefit to both the skeletal and cardiovascular systems (Goldman and Toteson, 1991; Lindsay, 1991). Yet one of the first questions many women ask, is 'Is there an alternative?'

For some women, the idea of taking hormones seems unnatural or unsafe. Others cannot take HRT because of known medical contraindications (see Chapter 6). Whether or not a woman considers HRT will depend partly on the severity of her symptoms and her own knowledge and perceptions of HRT. Some women will view HRT as a last resort, trying all other options first.

Others are very opposed to the principle of taking extra hormones at any time and so will not consider it at the time of menopause, however unpleasant their symptoms. For women such as these, alternative or complementary therapies may be useful.

This chapter discusses both conventional and complementary therapies and looks at how they may be useful for the woman with menopausal symptoms. Some are available through the National Health Service (NHS), whilst others require consultation with a specialist practitioner. It also discusses the importance of maintaining a healthy body throughout the climacteric, offering advice and tips on living a healthy lifestyle.

CONVENTIONAL DRUG THERAPY

HRT alleviates menopausal symptoms by treating the underlying cause – oestrogen deficiency. Nonhormonal therapies are aimed at alleviating individual symptoms.

Clonidine

Clonidine is a drug which was first used to treat migraine and has been found to be useful in reducing the intensity of hot flushes (Claydon et al, 1974; Edington et al, 1980). It is used for short periods (approximately 6 months) and then gradually stopped. The recommended dose for relief of hot flushes is 50 μg twice daily. Women should be warned of possible side-effects – dry mouth, dizziness and headaches, and advised not to discontinue the medication suddenly because of its hypotensive effects.

Antidepressants

Some would argue that there are few indications for the use of antidepressants in relieving mood changes which arise at the time of the menopause. It is true that clinical depression is not a typical menopausal symptom, although some may view the climacteric as a time of increased stress and strain. Some women may be depressed as well as menopausal, so careful evaluation by a sympathetic professional may be useful. Some women may also benefit from therapies such as counselling or psychotherapy as well as or instead of HRT.

Tranquillizers

Tranquillizers may be useful in times of extreme stress, such as bereavement, but are best avoided in the long term. The days when women in mid life were considered 'neurotic' and thus prescribed tranquillizers for their 'nerves' have, it is hoped, passed. Tranquillizers have not been shown to relieve vasomotor symptoms.

Vaginal lubricants

HRT is available as a local treatment for relief of vaginal symptoms. However for those women who wish to avoid hormones completely, alternatives are available. Traditional nonhormonal lubricants, such as KY Jelly, may assist in making intercourse less painful, but are not longlasting. Other lubricants include 'Senselle' which has a thinner consistency and which some women find easier to use. These are available over the counter from chemists. Water-based vaginal lubricants are recommended rather than oil-based ones such as baby oil or petroleum jelly.

A nonhormonal vaginal moisturizing gel is also available (Replens). This should be used on a regular basis (three times weekly), lowering the pH of the vagina and improving vaginal blood flow. Some women prefer to use this as it is not used in association with intercourse and yet is still nonhormonal.

DIETARY SUPPLEMENTS

Vitamin B6 (pyridoxine)

Some women experience more premenstrual symptoms during the perimenopause. Such symptoms may also occur with the use of cyclical HRT. Vitamin B6 is reported to be effective at reducing mood swings, breast tenderness and muscle aches, although some believe the benefits to be at least partly due to the placebo effect (Wilson, 1992).

A dose of 25–50 mg is suggested, either daily or 2 weeks premenstrually. Vitamin B6 can be purchased over the counter at chemists or health food shops. Vitamin B is present in green vegetables, nuts, seeds, brewers yeast and wholegrains.

Vitamin E

It is claimed that vitamin E may help relieve menopausal flushes but this is not verified by scientific studies. Fairly high doses would be required (800–1600 units a day) which some doctors are not in favour of because of potential long-term side-effects (Nachtigall and Rattner-Heilman, 1986). At a lower dose (400 units daily), vitamin E may help relieve breast tenderness (Wilson, 1992). Vitamin E is also available in oil form, which some claim will relieve vaginal dryness. Vitamin E is found in vegetable oils, cereals, dried beans and wholegrains.

Gamma linolenic acid (GLA)

GLA is found in Oil of Evening Primrose and in Starflower Oil. In some women it seems to help premenstrual symptoms such as breast tenderness. However studies have failed to demonstrate any greater benefit to menopausal flushes than a placebo (Chenoy et al, 1994).

Other minerals

There has been a marked increase in the number of supplements available to help women at the time of the menopause. They may contain magnesium, zinc, boron, potassium or other minerals. Whilst it is true that all of these minerals are an essential part of a healthy diet, it is unclear whether supplementing these minerals is of any clinical value in helping women through the climacteric years.

DRUG-FREE THERAPIES

Some women would prefer to see through the menopausal years in as natural a way as possible. This will mean avoiding all therapeutic drugs, not just HRT. The menopause is viewed as a transition, one which may impose temporary symptoms which are tolerated as much as possible without drugs. Women may seek medical advice for confirmation of their suspicions, but not seek medical intervention. Women who hold such beliefs may accept and benefit from forms of therapy which are perceived as more 'natural' and which do not involve the use of medication.

Relaxation

It is claimed that relaxation helps people deal with problems and conflicts in a calmer way (Wells and Tschudin, 1994). Some studies have shown that hot flushes can be reduced by behavioural relaxation methods (Germaine and Freedman, 1984; Freedman and Woodward, 1992). Slow deep breathing reduced flushes in small groups of women as an alternative to HRT. Learning to relax during a flush is not easy, but may help to diminish its intensity. Relaxation may also help women to cope with symptoms such as irritability, anxiety and panic attacks.

Methods of relaxation

- Focus your mind on a specific object or point, breathing in and out deeply, slowly and evenly, concentrating on the object in mind.
- Gradually tense then relax every muscle group of the body in sequence, perhaps starting at the top of the body and working down, or at the periphery (fingers and toes) and working in.
- Concentrate your mind on a visual scene which you find relaxing and pleasant, breathing deeply as you do so. Remind yourself to keep your facial muscles relaxed.

NONHORMONAL MANAGEMENT
— Drug-free therapies

Stress reduction

Stress is a normal experience. Recognizing and coping with stress becomes a regular part of our modern day lives. Some degree of stress is beneficial – it keeps us going at our jobs, it may help to improve performance and presents us with challenges, which when conquered, give us a tremendous sense of achievement. Each of us has a certain point at which individual stressors become unmanageable and which may lead to difficulties, either physically, psychologically or emotionally. The key to reducing stress is to understand your own abilities, ambitions and weaknesses and to recognize when you are moving beyond that which is bearable (Wilson, 1992).

The perimenopausal years may be particularly stressful for some women. Change in itself is a stress factor and for some women, there will be a number of changes in their life at this time. Such changes may be:

- Children leaving home
- Bereavement
- Financial difficulties
- Marriage difficulties
- Changes in health

It is important to learn to deal with stress whilst, in the long term, finding a way of solving the stressful situation itself. Sometimes, menopausal symptoms can themselves be a cause of stress and anxiety, particulary if they cause disruption to the normal living pattern.

Suggested ways of alleviating stress are:

- Relaxation/visualization
- Exercise
- Meditation
- Yoga
- Flotation therapy
- Acupuncture
- Shiatsu

Counselling

For some women, the menopause occurs just at the time when life's pressures may seem to be the greatest. Physical and psychological symptoms may lead to a woman feeling less able to cope with the particular stresses in her life, which ordinarily she would cope with well. Minor anxieties can become major concerns. Some women are less able to cope with problems when physically tired or less able to deal with a relationship when they feel under pressure because of psychological symptoms, such as mood swings, irritability or poor memory.

A counsellor may help a woman to face issues which have remained hidden, but which are highlighted by the implications of the menopause. The menopause itself can be viewed as a life event, which prompts some women to re-evaluate the life they live. Areas in which a woman may benefit from the help of a counsellor include:

- Marital/relationship problems
- Facing childlessness
- Work-related anxiety
- Health worries
- Longstanding unresolved problems

Support groups

Some women value the opportunity to discuss their problems with others who can identify with how they are feeling. It can be reassuring to learn that other women are experiencing similar feelings or symptoms. Women may feel isolated during the time of the climacteric, considering that what they are experiencing is unusual, simply because they have not discussed the issue with other women. Simply learning that other women are in the same situation can be reassuring. For more details about running a support group see Chapter 9.

ALTERNATIVE/COMPLEMENTARY THERAPIES

Alternative or complementary therapies are so-called because they do not embrace 'orthodox' medicine, by an 'orthodox' medical practitioner. The term alternative conveys the idea of a parallel but independent system of therapy. It often refers to unconventional methods which have not been subjected to scientific review or clinical trials. Some practitioners prefer the term complementary implying that such therapies may be used as an adjunct to conventional medicine as well as instead of it (Sharma, 1992).

Training

Training in complementary therapies varies enormously even within one therapy area, but also between therapies. It is important to choose a therapist carefully and to ensure that they are working within approved guidelines in their chosen therapy area. Most complementary therapies have their own representative body which will offer advice on choosing a therapist. Some hold a register o" therapists who have a particular level of training or qua lification.

Homeopathy – *'Like cures like'*

Homeopathy works on the principle that a substance which is poisonous in large doses can cure when used in very small doses (Scott and Scott, 1991). In other words, if the symptoms produced by large, harmful quantities of the substance are the same as those produced by a particular illness then homeopathy can cure that illness. The

Table 8.1   Suggested homeopathic remedies for menopausal symptoms (Smith, 1984)

Remedy	Symptom
Lachesis	Hot flushes
Pulsatilla	
Calendula	Vaginal dryness
Bryonia	
Sepia	Loss of libido, irritability

amount of substance used in homeopathy will be very small and very dilute.

Preparations

Homeopathic remedies originate from animal, mineral or herbal matter, often prepared in alcohol and diluted many times. At each dilution the flask containing the liquid is subjected to strong agitation, by banging or shaking. This is believed to spread the remedy's energy through the preparation. Remedies are usually sold in the form of tablets, capsules, powder or liquid. Whilst taking a homeopathic remedy the user is advised to avoid coffee or peppermint (including peppermint toothpaste) as these may negate the remedy's effects. Some homeopathic remedies are available from healthfood stores but a recognized practitioner will try to tailor the treatment to a woman's needs.

Effect on menopausal symptoms

As yet there are no scientific data to support the value of homeopathic medicine in relieving acute menopausal symptoms (Ullman, 1991; Bayley, 1993). However individual women may find it effective.

Acupuncture – 'to pierce with a needle'

Acupuncture originated in China and is one of many traditional medicines practised in China today. Others include herbal medicine, massage and dietary therapy. In China, such traditional therapies have been widely used and are now fully integrated into the Chinese Health Service alongside Western medicine (Hillier and Jewell, 1983).

Acupuncture has been practised on a large scale in the UK for 25 years or more (Wells and Tschudin, 1994). The theory of acupuncture is that good health is essentially the result of a healthy internal environment. Life energy forces are believed to flow through the body along channels or meridians. Acupuncture reportedly restores the flow of energy using copper, silver or gold needles which

NONHORMONAL MANAGEMENT – Alternative/ complementary therapies

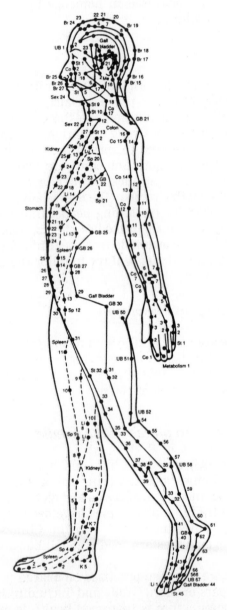

Figure 8.1   Acupuncture – a traditional Chinese medicine.

Table 8.2 Herbs suggested for relief of menopausal symptoms

Herb	Symptom
Yarrow	Hot flushes
Mexican Yam	Hot flushes, loss of energy
Ginseng	Loss of libido, vaginal dryness
Schizandra	Irritability, insomnia

are inserted into the skin or underlying tissues. The points of needle insertion are decided by the practitioner according to the channels and systems which he/she considers to need improvement.

Effect on menopausal symptoms

Scientific evidence is lacking with regard to the use of acupuncture and menopausal symptoms. However a small study in Sweden demonstrated a significant reduction in the number of hot flushes experienced by women treated with electrostimulated acupuncture – an improvement which was maintained 3 months later. Large-scale studies are not available.

Herbal therapy

Herbs and plants have been used for healing for many centuries; indeed, many modern day medications were originally derived from plants. Herbal medicine uses small amounts of herbs, which when properly prepared are reported to contain the life force or 'vibration' of the plant. Modern herbalism aims to help the body correct itself by strengthening its natural functions so that it may heal itself (Scott and Scott, 1991).

Herbal remedies may be taken in the following ways:

* **Decoction** – dried herb is simmered in water for 10–30 minutes. The solids are discarded and the liquid retained.

NONHORMONAL MANAGEMENT – Alternative/ complementary therapies

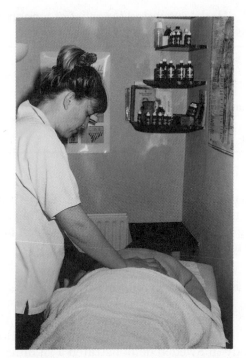

Figure 8.2   Aromatherapy – the use of essential oils. Reproduced with permission of Alison Campbell, Beauty Therapist. (Photograph by Mark Abernethy.)

- **Tincture** – Herb extract is soaked in a mixture of water and alcohol (ethyl alcohol). This mixture is diluted as necessary.

Side-effects are few with herbal medicine but a few people may be sensitive or allergic to specific herbs. Some herbs should be avoided in pregnancy.

Effect on menopausal symptoms

Many women have reported satisfaction with herbal remedies, although no clinical trials have been reported evaluating herbs as a means of alleviating menopausal symptoms. Some herbal remedies, such as Ginseng or Dong Quai are known to contain oestrogen-like substances. When used in large amounts, they have been shown to produce vaginal bleeding (Greenspan, 1983).

Aromatherapy

The way to health is to have an aromatic bath and scented massage every day.   Hippocrates.

Aromatherapy uses essential oils of plants in a controlled way to achieve balance and harmony in the human mind, body and spirit (Wells and Tschudin, 1994). These oils are either inhaled as a vapour or massaged through the skin. A professional aromatherapist will choose a blend of oils that will be individually tailored to their client's needs.

Although often considered to be an upmarket beauty treatment, aromatherapy is beginning to be recognized as having therapeutic value. Certainly a professional massage, combined with a sensitive therapist and pleasant aromas, must make the therapy of at least psychological benefit.

Effect on menopausal symptoms

Aromatherapists do not make claims of clinical improvements but rather of an improved sense of wellbeing among their clients. It is certainly possible that something which makes a woman feel less pressured and more relaxed could improve wellbeing at the time of the menopause.

There will always be some women who, for whatever reason, do not wish to take hormone replacement therapy. It is important to have at least some information about alternatives, so that women know where to turn to for more expert advice. You may not feel able to recommend a particular therapist, but can at least introduce some of the therapies into a woman's mind, leaving her to decide whether or not to pursue any of them. There has been a tendency for those advising women at the time of menopause to dismiss therapies other than HRT, simply because of lack of scientific evidence. As with all therapies, at the end of the day, the client will choose that which she finds most suitable.

NONHORMONAL MANAGEMENT – Alternative/ complementary therapies

LIVING A HEALTHY LIFESTYLE

Most women want to look good and feel fit all through their lives. For some reason the menopause is sometimes perceived as being the 'beginning of the end' as far as health and beauty are concerned, with the actual menopause marking the end of femininity and the beginning of old age. This is, of course, untrue – for some women the menopause occurs almost unnoticed. Some women, however, see the onset of menopause in a particularly positive way and consider it to be a time of transition into a new phase of life – a step in a new direction. This may make a woman re-evaluate her life, both physically and socially. The time of menopause may be the time which prompts a woman into thinking 'now is the time to make those health changes I have been promising myself. Now is the time to prepare for old age'.

A healthy lifestyle is to be commended at all ages Women often find themselves the targets of advice abou diet, exercise and lifestyle, so much so that they can feel pressurized into conforming to an image of health, beauty and fitness. Unfortunately many of the media messages about healthy living are accompanied by pictures of women who are not only unhealthily thin, but also very young. Women may feel that it is too late to make worthwhile changes in mid life, when in fact developing a healthier lifestyle at this age is still tremendously worthwhile.

Exercise

Women generally exercise less than men, yet exercise is important to the female body at all ages. It is vital for maintenance of strength, suppleness and stamina. Lack of exercise leads to increased bone loss and a deterioration in the cardiovascular system. When advising a woman about exercise it is important to consider her individual needs and physical condition. A woman in her fifties who has never exercised should be advised to build up her exercise gradually rather than embarking on a vigorous exercise programme straight away. If in doubt about her fitness, she should be advised to consult her doctor before commencing a new exercise programme.

Weight-bearing exercise, such as walking or dancing is best for helping to maintain bone density. The benefits of brisk walking are often underestimated. Swimming is an excellent exercise for improving stamina and maintaining suppleness of joints and muscles. Many women also gain benefit from anaerobic exercise such as body conditioning or stretching exercises. These are aimed at keeping the muscles toned and the figure trim.

As well as the physical benefits of regular exercise, some women describe the following:

- An increased sense of wellbeing
- A greater degree of self-confidence
- A sense of achievement and satisfaction
- Improved sleep pattern
- Reduction in anxiety levels

Diet

A healthy diet is always to be recommended. Most people understand the concepts of a healthy diet, but find it difficult to maintain over a long period. General recommendations for a healthy diet are:

- Reduction in total fat intake
- Reduction in salt intake
- Reduction of sugar intake
- Increased intake of starches and cereals
- Increased fibre intake

Perimenopausal women may need to be reminded of the importance of maintaining an adequate calcium intake, for the maintenance of healthy bone. There is some controversy over exactly how much calcium is required by a perimenopausal woman, but a recommendation of around 1000 mg is often made. Calcium is most easily obtained from dairy products but is also found in:

- Green vegetables
- Sardines
- Skimmed milk powder
- Figs

NONHORMONAL MANAGEMENT – Living a healthy lifestyle

WEIGHT (Stones and Pounds)

— 17 st
— 7 lbs
— 16 st
— 7 lbs
— 15 st
— 7 lbs
— 14 st
— 7 lbs
— 13 st
— 7 lbs
— 12 st
— 7 lbs

HEIGHT (Feet and Inches)

WEIGHT (Kilograms)

WEIGHT (Stones and Pounds): 11 st — 7 lbs — 10 st — 7 lbs — 9 st — 7 lbs — 8 st — 7 lbs — 7 st

WEIGHT (Kilograms)	1.36		1.40		1.44		1.48		1.52		1.56		1.60		1.64		1.68		1.72		1.76		1.80		1.84		1.88		1.92		1.96		2.00
71	38	37	36	35	34	33	32	32	31	30	29	28	28	27	26	26	25	25	24	23	23	22	22	21	21	21	20	20	19	19	18	18	18
70	38	37	36	35	34	33	32	31	30	30	29	28	27	27	26	25	25	24	24	23	23	22	22	21	21	20	20	19	19	19	18	18	17
69	37	36	35	34	33	32	32	31	30	29	28	28	27	26	26	25	24	24	23	23	22	22	21	21	20	20	20	19	19	18	18	18	17
68	37	36	35	34	33	32	31	30	29	29	28	27	27	26	25	25	24	24	23	22	22	21	21	21	20	20	19	19	18	18	18	17	17
67	36	35	34	33	32	31	31	30	29	28	28	27	26	26	25	24	24	23	23	22	22	21	21	20	20	19	19	19	18	18	17	17	17
66	36	35	34	33	32	31	30	29	29	28	27	26	26	25	25	24	23	23	22	22	21	21	20	20	19	19	19	18	18	18	17	17	16
65	35	34	33	32	31	30	30	29	28	27	27	26	25	25	24	24	23	22	22	21	21	21	20	20	19	19	18	18	18	17	17	17	16
64	35	34	33	32	31	30	29	28	28	27	26	26	25	24	24	23	23	22	22	21	21	20	20	19	19	18	18	18	17	17	17	16	16
63	34	33	32	31	30	30	29	28	27	27	26	25	25	24	23	23	22	22	21	21	20	20	19	19	19	18	18	17	17	17	16	16	16
62	34	33	32	31	30	29	28	28	27	26	25	25	24	24	23	22	22	21	21	20	20	20	19	19	18	18	18	17	17	16	16	16	15
61	33	32	31	30	29	29	28	27	26	26	25	24	24	23	23	22	22	21	21	20	20	19	19	18	18	18	17	17	17	16	16	16	15
60	32	32	31	30	29	28	27	27	26	25	25	24	23	23	22	22	21	21	20	20	19	19	19	18	18	17	17	17	16	16	16	15	15
59	32	31	30	29	28	28	27	26	26	25	24	24	23	22	22	21	21	20	20	19	19	19	18	18	17	17	17	16	16	16	15	15	15
58	31	30	30	29	28	27	26	26	25	24	24	23	23	22	22	21	21	20	20	19	19	18	18	18	17	17	16	16	16	15	15	15	14
57	31	30	29	28	27	27	26	25	25	24	23	23	22	22	21	21	20	20	19	19	18	18	18	17	17	16	16	16	15	15	15	15	14
56	30	29	29	28	27	26	26	25	24	24	23	22	22	21	21	20	20	19	19	18	18	18	17	17	17	16	16	16	15	15	15	14	14
55	30	29	28	27	27	26	25	24	24	23	23	22	21	21	20	20	19	19	19	18	18	17	17	17	16	16	16	15	15	15	14	14	14
54	29	28	28	27	26	25	25	24	23	23	22	22	21	21	20	20	19	19	18	18	17	17	17	16	16	16	15	15	15	14	14	14	13
53	29	28	27	26	26	25	24	24	23	22	22	21	21	20	20	19	19	18	18	18	17	17	16	16	16	15	15	15	14	14	14	14	13
52	28	27	27	26	25	24	24	23	23	22	21	21	20	20	19	19	18	18	18	17	17	16	16	16	15	15	15	14	14	14	14	13	13
51	28	27	26	25	25	24	23	23	22	22	21	20	20	19	19	19	18	18	17	17	16	16	16	15	15	15	14	14	14	14	13	13	13
50	27	26	26	25	24	23	23	22	22	21	21	20	20	19	19	18	18	17	17	17	16	16	15	15	15	14	14	14	14	13	13	13	12
49	26	26	25	24	24	23	22	22	21	21	20	20	19	19	18	18	17	17	17	16	16	15	15	15	14	14	14	14	13	13	13	12	12
48	26	25	24	24	23	23	22	21	21	20	20	19	19	18	18	17	17	17	16	16	15	15	15	14	14	14	14	13	13	13	12	12	12
47	25	25	24	23	23	22	21	21	20	20	19	19	18	18	17	17	17	16	16	16	15	15	15	14	14	14	13	13	13	12	12	12	12
46	25	24	23	23	22	22	21	20	20	19	19	18	18	18	17	17	16	16	16	15	15	15	14	14	14	13	13	13	12	12	12	12	11
45	24	24	23	22	22	21	21	20	19	19	18	18	18	17	17	16	16	16	15	15	15	14	14	14	13	13	13	12	12	12	12	11	11
44	24	23	22	22	21	21	20	20	19	19	18	18	17	17	16	16	16	15	15	15	14	14	14	13	13	13	12	12	12	12	11	11	11

HEIGHT (Metres)

Very Obese
Health is seriously at risk. Losing weight **immediately** is essential.

Obese
Health is at risk. Losing weight **now** should be seriously considered.

Overweight
Health could suffer. Some weight loss should now be considered.

Healthy
A desirable BMI figure indicating a healthy weight.

Underweight

Figure 8.3 Body mass index – a guide to ideal weight.

Whilst most women will take sufficient calcium through their diet, some may need calcium supplementation, particularly if they have a restricted diet, perhaps for religious or moral reasons. Such women are advised to discuss the issue with their doctor rather than simply buying supplements of their own accord.

Many women complain of weight gain around the time of the menopause. Certainly as women age, the metabolic rate changes and women who continue to consume the same number of calories will gain weight unless they also increase their calorie requirements through exercise. Some women reduce their intake of dairy produce in an attempt to eliminate fats, thereby losing a valuable source of calcium. It would be more beneficial to use low fat milk, which contains as much calcium as full fat milk, without compromising on fat intake.

Alcohol

The recommendation from the Department of Health is that women should restrict their alcohol intake to 21 units per week. Excessive alcohol inhibits calcium absorption and is also known to reduce osteoblastic activity, thus increasing the risk of osteoporosis. One unit of alcohol is equivalent to:

• Half a pint of beer, lager or cider
• Single glass of wine
• Single pub measure of port, sherry or spirits, such as vodka and whisky

Smoking

Overall, there has been a decline in smoking in the UK, but it appears that women are less likely than men to give up. At a younger age, they are also more likely to start smoking than boys (Westcott, 1994). Research has shown that smokers are aware of the reasons that they should stop, yet the anti-smoking advice is often ignored (Graham, 1993). Smoking is particularly relevant to women, because apart from the risk factors of smoking associated with both men and women, it has an adverse effect on the two body systems already profoundly affected by hormone changes at the time of the menopause – the cardiovascular system and the skeleton. It therefore makes complete sense to encourage a woman to quit smoking at this time of her life.

It is recognized, however, that quitting smoking is not easy – 70% of people who are trying to stop, smoke again within 3 months (Benowitz, 1988). Women, in particular, may be concerned about gaining weight if they stop smoking. Sensitive counselling and personal support are an essential part of advising a woman to stop smoking.

NOT SIMPLY HORMONES...

Although physiologically, the menopause represents a single event relating to a woman's hormones, we have come to use the term 'menopause' in a wider sense. There is a danger that we fail to look at the whole woman and concentrate only correcting her imbalanced hormones. Women themselves are demanding much more than this, wanting advice on a whole range of issues relating to mid life. This will encompass all aspects of healthy living, as well as responding to the need for information about HRT or other treatments for menopausal symptoms.

REFERENCES

Bayley C (1993) Homeopathy. *J. Med. Philo*s. **18**(2): 129–145.

Benowitz NL (1988) Pharmacologic aspects of cigarette smoking and nicotine addiction. *N. Engl. J. Med.* **319**: 1318–1330.

Chenoy R, Hussein S, Tayob Y et al (1994) Effect of gamolenic acid from evening primrose oil on menopausal flushing. *Br. Med. J.* **308**: 501–503.

Claydon JR, Bell JW & Pollard P (1974) Menopausal flushing. Double blind trial of a non hormonal preparation. *Br. Med. J.* **1**: 409.

Coope J, Thompson JM & Poller L (1975) Effects of 'natural oestrogen' replacement therapy on menopausal symptoms and blood clotting. *Br. Med. J.* **4**: 139–143.

Dennerstein L (1988) Psychiatric aspects of the climacteric. In Studd JWW & Whitehead MI (eds) *The Menopause*, pp. 43–54. Oxford: Blackwell Scientific.

Edington RF, Chagnon JP & Steinberg WM (1980) Clonidine for menopausal flushing. *Can. Med. Assoc. J.* **123**: 23.

Freedman RR & Woodward S (1992) Behavioural treatment of menopausal hot flushes: evaluation by ambulatory monitoring. *Am. J. Obstet. Gynecol.* **167**: 436–439.

Germaine LM & Freedman RR (1984) Behavioural treatment of hot flushes: Evaluation of objective methods. *J. Consult. Clin. Psychol.* **52**: 1072–1079.

Goldman L & Toteson AN (1991) Uncertainty about postmenopausal oestrogen. *N. Engl. J. Med.* **325**(11): 800–802.

Graham H (1993) Women's smoking: Government targets and social trends. *Health Visitor* **66**(3): 80–82.

Greenspan EM (1983) Ginseng and vaginal bleeding. *J. Am. Med. Assoc.* **249**: 2018.

Hillier SM & Jewell JA (1983) *Health Care and Traditional Medicine in China 1800–1982*. London: Routledge.

Hunt K (1988) Perceived value of treatment among a group of long term users of HRT. *J.R. Coll. Gen. Pract.* **38**: 389–401.

Lindsay R (1991) Estrogens, bone mass and osteoporotic fracture. *Am. J. Med.* **91**(Suppl. 5b): 10s–13s.

Nachtigall L & Rattner-Heilman J (1986) *Estrogen: The facts can change your life*. Los Angeles, USA: The Body Press.

Scott J & Scott S (1991) *Natural Medicine for Women*. Gaia Books Ltd.

Sharma U (1992) *Complementary Medicine Today – Practitioners and Patients*. London: Routledge.

Smith T (1984) *A Woman's Guide to Homeopathic Medicine*. Wellingborough, UK: Thorsons.

Ullman D (1991) *Discovering Homeopathy: Medicine for the 21st Century*. North Atlantic Books.

Wells R & Tschudin V (eds) (1994) *Well's Supportive Therapies in Health Care*. London: Balliere Tindall.

Westcott P (1994) *Women's Health*. London, Nursing Times/ Macmillan.

Wilson RCD (1992) *Understanding HRT and the Menopause*. London: Consumers Association.

Chapter 9

Patient Support

It is acknowledged that HRT offers women relief from menopausal symptoms as well as conferring long-term benefits to the skeletal and cardiovascular system. It has been suggested that it should be offered to many more than the estimated 10–20% of women who currently take it in the UK (Belchetz, 1989). Yet despite an enormous interest in the subject of menopause, many women still do not fully understand the changes that occur in their bodies at this time (NOP, 1991; Hope and Rees, 1995). One study showed that of over 1000 women questioned, two-thirds did not recognize that the menopause was caused by the ovaries ceasing to function (NOP, 1991). Other studies have shown that women often have a poor knowledge of the consequences of oestrogen deficiency and therefore do not know the potentially beneficial effects of HRT (Sinclair et al, 1993).

So do British women refuse HRT because of known risks and expected side-effects, or are they simply unaware of the availability of HRT and therefore do not request it? In Scotland, a study showed that of the 1100 women surveyed, many had experienced menopausal symptoms for over 6 months, yet 70% had not even considered HRT and nearly 80% had not discussed the matter with a doctor (Sinclair et al, 1993). Most women want more information, not just about HRT, but also about the menopause itself (Draper and Roland, 1990; Roberts, 1991). Such information is surely most useful to a woman before the menopause, to prepare her for what is to come and to allow her time to consider all the facts as they apply to her circumstances.

This chapter suggests ways of providing the information necessary for a woman to decide for herself whether HRT is appropriate. Certainly some women will choose not to take HRT, but let us ensure that their decision is based on accurate facts and not assumptions and myths; this, then, is truly an 'informed choice'. The chapter also contains questions which are commonly asked by women about hormone replacement therapy. Reading them will help increase you awareness of potential concerns and also broaden your knowledge of the subject.

DECISION-MAKING

Unlike may areas of medicine, the advice about whether to take HRT is often not clear cut – it is appropriate for some women and not for others. You cannot simply advise a woman that she would be foolish to refuse HRT, as you might advise a diabetic who needs insulin. With a condition such as diabetes, the facts are clear-cut and the consequences of not taking insulin profound. In the area of HRT, you may need to spend a great deal of time discussing perceived risks and benefits as they apply to the individual woman concerned. We talk about helping a woman to make 'an informed choice' about HRT, rather than simply telling her what to do. Sometimes it can be hard to allow a woman to make her choice, which may not be that which you would recommend. Yet women themselves expect to do just that – to gather information and then to make their own choice. There are well known risks and benefits to taking HRT, but the decision to take it is a complex one, requiring input and consideration from the individual as well as from the health professional. It is not enough to simply advise a women, we must encourage her to take a decision and then be prepared to help her carry it through.

Rothert states that there are three main factors involved in making a decision about HRT:

- Base rate risks
- Perceived personal risk
- Personal values

In helping women decide about HRT you can inform them of the base rate risk (e.g. of breast cancer), assist them to assess their personal risk (for example of osteoporosis), whilst helping them acknowledge their personal values (Rothert et al, 1990).

Base rate risks relate to known facts, such as the incidence of osteoporosis or coronary heart disease after the menopause, the benefits of HRT and possible side-effects. These are common to all women and should be provided as background information to making a decision.

Perceived personal risk is influenced by actual experiences. Two women with identical medical backgrounds may perceive their personal risk in different ways. As health professionals we help to quantify the personal risk by making an assessment of risk factors, for example of heart disease or osteoporosis. Helping women to identify their risks enables them to make a suitable choice.

Personal values describe what is important to an individual woman. For example, some women are more concerned about breast cancer than heart disease. These women would be cautious about taking any medication which might increase their risk of breast disease, however small the risk. Other women are more worried about strokes or heart attacks and are prepared to take a risk on the breast cancer issue. Some women consider the use of any hormones to be unnatural, others are not concerned about this issue. Personal values cannot be wrong and will vary from woman to woman. Any decision about HRT must be consistent with a woman's personal values if she is to persevere with the decision she has made.

SOURCES OF INFORMATION

Media

The subject of 'the change', and in particular HRT, is very popular with the press. Women's magazines, radio programmes and daily newspapers have all covered some aspect of the subject over the last few years – some with greater accuracy than others. Women themselves seem to find such articles very useful and many say that they are the main source of information after their General Practitioner (NOP, 1991). Sadly in some parts of the country, women have valued the media as a source of information, more than the practice nurse (NOP, 1991). Hopefully, as practice nurses become more widely accepted and respected as an integral part of the primary healthcare team, these views will change.

Health professionals working in the field of menopause should try to keep up-to-date with media messages about HRT. Women may come to you to discuss such issues and it is helpful if you are aware of the

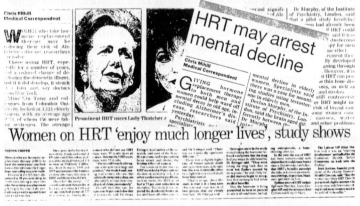

Figure 9.1   Headlines showing positive messages are often forgotten. (*Independent*, 3rd Jan. 1996; *Guardian*, 10th Jul. 1996, 16th Aug. 1996.)

views expressed. Some articles are excellent and may be worth keeping as a resource, whilst others concentrate only on the perceived 'youth effects' of HRT, or highlight the frightening stores relating to HRT use.

Primary healthcare team

Most women who experience menopausal symptoms do not need referral to a hospital clinic. General practitioners (GP) can expertly treat and advise women, referring women to a specialist clinic only when necessary. However women often express a general dissatisfaction with the advice received from their GP and some will travel many miles to be seen in a specialist clinic (Garnett et al, 1991).

This may be because consultation times with GPs are too brief to cover adequately all aspects of the menopause and HRT. One survey revealed that the average GP consultation for menopause-related issues was 10 minutes, compared to 45 minutes with a specialist (Amarant Trust Survey, 1992). Eighty percent of women questioned expressed dissatisfaction at this. Not surprisingly, women look elsewhere for accurate information. In response, some practices are recognizing the problem and seeking ways of providing information outside of general consultations with the GP. Practice nurses are becoming more involved in informing women about HRT and the menopause. A survey of 800 practice nurses showed that 76% of practices were running a well woman clinic, most providing some advice on the subject of menopause. In many practices, the role was shared equally between GPs and nurses, with a common pattern of care beginning with an assessment of a woman by the GP who initiates therapy. After this the nurse counsels the woman on her chosen treatment and offers general lifestyle advice. Yet 61% of the nurses surveyed identified a need for management protocols and 80% of respondents said they needed more training (Shine, 1995). These issues need to be addressed before practice nurses can be expected to take on a greater role in menopause counselling.

Training

There is no nationally recognized course (such as there is with family planning), dedicated to the subject of menopause and HRT, either for doctors or nurses. For doctors, training is usually through approved courses and study days as part of general post-basic education. Nurse training in menopause varies around the country with some areas offering local courses, whilst other areas of the country have very little in terms of training. Organizations such as the Amarant Trust, the National Osteoporosis Society, the British Menopause Society and Women's Health Concern have all organized study days for nurses and doctors on the subject of menopause and HRT. Some local specialist menopause clinics organize occasional study days. Finally, pharmaceutical companies offer training and support for health professionals wanting to learn more about HRT.

Table 9.1   Suggested roles and responsibilities

Nurse	Doctor
Initial identification of patients	Review suitability for HRT
Information and advice	Physical examination
Menopause	Secondary investigations
HRT	Initiate treatment
Lifestyle	6-Month check
Assessment for HRT	Change treatment if necessary
3-Month check	Regular checks – alternating
Regular checks – alternating	with nurse
with GP	
Be available to women for ongoing	
advice (telephone)	
Discussion of nonhormonal	
alternatives	
Identify problems and refer to GP	

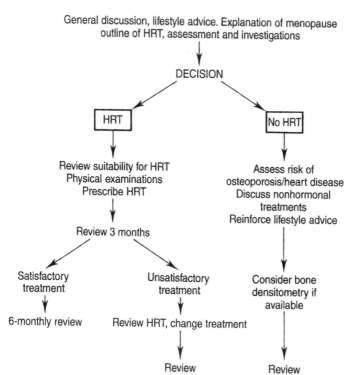

General discussion, lifestyle advice. Explanation of menopause
outline of HRT, assessment and investigations

↓

DECISION

HRT   No HRT

Review suitability for HRT
Physical examinations
Prescribe HRT

↓

Review 3 months

Satisfactory treatment   Unsatisfactory treatment   Consider bone densitometry if available

6-monthly review   Review HRT, change treatment

Review   Review

Assess risk of
osteoporosis/heart disease
Discuss nonhormonal
treatments
Reinforce lifestyle advice

Figure 9.2   **Suggested management plan for new patients.**

Protocols

Defining a protocol of care will ensure that every woman receives the same high level of individual advice and assessment, whichever health professional they see. It also means that within a team, each member knows what is expected and performs their role accordingly. It is important to define the care which can be taken on by the practice nurse and that which the doctor should perform. These roles and responsibilities will vary according to the training and competence of the nurse and the support and encouragement offered by the GP. Table 9.1 suggests how responsibilities may be divided. There will usually be a degree of overlap where it is agreed that either the nurse or doctor are appropriate.

PATIENT SUPPORT
– Sources of information

MENOPAUSE CLINIC PROTOCOL

Take an accurate personal and medical history, taking note of risk factors, contraindications and symptoms.

Name _____ Dob _____ NHS No _____ Address _____

Date of menopause _____ Age at menopause _____

Medical history

family history of CVD _____ liver disease _____
thrombosis _____ DVT _____
hypertension _____ gallstones _____
migraine _____ otosclerosis _____
history of cancer _____ cholecystectomy _____
mastectomy _____ varicose veins _____
breast disease _____ epilepsy _____
breast lumps _____ fibroids _____
diabetes _____ endometrial hyperplasia _____
hysterectomy _____
oophorectomy _____
endometriosis _____
other medications _____

Gynaecological history

menstrual history _____
last menstrual period _____
irregularity _____
PCB _____
IMB _____
PMB _____
amenorrhoea _____
PMT _____
contraception _____
parity _____

Psychological history

Date

depression _____
anxiety _____
other _____

Social

problems at home or work _____
smoking:
no of cigarettes per day _____
alcohol:
no of units per week _____
exercise (outdoor) _____
diet _____

Menopausal symptoms

Hot flushes/palpitations............ ☐   Irritability/loss of confidence........... ☐   Urinary symptoms/prolapse........ ☐   Joint pains/backache........

Night sweats/insomnia............ ☐   Vaginal dryness/dyspareunia.......... ☐   Depression/loss of libido............ ☐   Fatigue........

Risk factors for osteoporosis

Investigations	Breast exam (1yr)	Pelvic exam (1yr)	Cervical smear (3yrs)	Mammography (3yrs)
Date/result				
Date/result				
Date/result				
Date/result				

family history

previous history

drug history

Examination and investigation

Date	Weight	Height	Blood pressure	Urine	Fasting lipids	FSH/LH levels (if necessary)	Haemoglobin (if necessary)	Thyroid function (if necessary)	HRT

Counselling
Inform the patient about the causes and symptoms of the menopause, options for treatment, life-style changes, advice on contraception and details of helpline

Follow-up
Assessment at four to six weeks after first appointment and at 3-6 month intervals thereafter. Check bleeding patterns, side-effects and any other problems

Figure 9.3 Typical patient history sheet. From 'The Menopause and HRT – A practice nurse's guide' by F. Symes, from The Prescriber, with permission.

Providing information

Once it is recognized that a 10-minute consultation is insufficient for providing adequate information about HRT and menopause, you can choose the method which is appropriate for your situation. Some doctors rely on the nurse to provide the basic information, whilst others will work together to help women come to a decision. The following may be helpful:

Group sessions. Some practice nurses have organized regular meetings to which women are invited to come to hear about the subject of menopause and HRT. During the session, general information about menopause and HRT is provided, outlining basic physiology, an introduction to HRT and some information about the long-term consequences of oestrogen deficiency. It is not designed to meet all individuals needs and women are invited to make a personal consultation with their doctor or practice nurse if appropriate. However, it does mean that when a woman attends for her consultation, she will already have the basic knowledge needed to ask relevant questions and perhaps to make a decision for herself. For the nurse or general practitioner, this is a valuable use of time and for the women themselves, it means that they probably get more time spent on information giving and questions than would otherwise be the case.

Sometimes these meetings are open to any women who are interested, others are by invitation, targetting certain women, perhaps by age, or by medical history (e.g. hysterectomized women, or those using corticosteroid therapy).

A disadvantage of this type of group is that some women may overwhelm the meeting and others may get a distorted view of HRT from any individuals who have not found a suitable type for themselves. Another drawback is that for some women, group meetings can be very threatening, particularly if they consider the menopause to be a personal issue. The very people who need the information may not come at all. Other women will be very grateful for the opportunity to discuss the issue without feeling an obligation to at least try HRT if that seems to be what the nurse or doctor recommends. A group meeting can be suitably anonymous for those who want it to be! If you are in an area with a high population of a particular ethnic group you may consider holding an information evening specifically for them, involving a community representative and translator if necessary, taking into account the needs of that particular ethnic group.

Some practices have put together a complete programme of meetings over about 6 weeks, covering issues such as: What is the menopause?, lifestyle issues at mid life, well woman care, HRT, osteoporosis, heart disease, sexuality and relationships, alternative therapies. These meetings may be organized in conjunction with several health professionals, including practice nurses, health visitors, family planning nurses, pharmacists, GPs and dieticians.

Support groups.   Support groups differ from group information meetings in that support group members are encouraged to feel comfortable enough to talk in a safe, supportive environment. There may be a health professional present, but the women themselves often lead or contribute to the meeting. It can be encouraging for a woman who is suffering symptoms to discover that what she is experiencing is not unusual. A woman can feel isolated, particularly if she is younger than average and she may feel unable to express her concerns to friends or family. Meeting women in a similar situation can be very useful.

Guidelines for leading a support group are:

- Choose your venue, making it easily accessible, welcoming and comfortable
- Introduce yourself and state the purpose of the group
- Keep discussion going, asking leading questions and inviting people to contribute
- Be prepared for a dominant group member, redirecting the discussion if necessary
- Be aware of the time, finishing promptly
- Review the group regularly

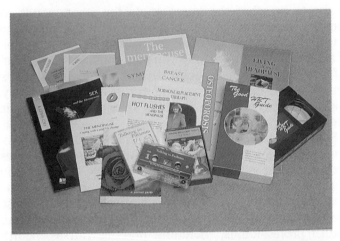

Figure 9.4   Various literature. (Courtesy of the Medical Illustration Department, Northwick Park Institute for Medical Research, Northwick Park Hospital, Harrow, Middlesex.)

Individual targetting. You may consider that it is most important to aim your information at those women who are known to have risk factors for osteoporosis or heart disease. If you have computerized records, you will be able to decide on certain risk factors and individually target women with those risks. Risk factors you may include would be:

- Early menopause
- Early hysterectomy
- Prolonged use of corticosteroid therapy
- Strong family history of heart disease
- Women who have already experienced one fracture since the age of 40 years
- Episodes of amenorrhoea in the past (unrelated to pregnancy)
- History of anorexia nervosa

This method has the advantage of reaching those women who are most likely to benefit from HRT and the information can be related specifically at the risk factors involved. Women who are invited may be more likely to attend than with an open invitation, but it is important to be sure that women are not frightened by the thought that they have been targetted as a possible candidate for a disease.

Literature. Having good quality literature available for women to take away means that women can read at their own pace, share the information with their partners or friends and return for discussion when they feel it is appropriate. Leaflets can be useful in that they are often provided free of charge to clinics and are unbiased towards any particular product, even though they are often provided by the pharmaceutical industry. However, they are usually strongly in favour of the use of HRT as opposed to trying alternative ways of relieving symptoms. They rightly stress the benefits of long-term HRT which can be useful for some women. Such literature should be used in addition to a full and frank discussion and not instead of it. Literature can also be obtained from some of the health charities and organizations listed elsewhere in this chapter, but there may be a nominal charge for them. Some authorities have health promotion units which will act as a resource centre and give guidance about what may be available. Literature is available in languages other than English for those who need it.

Videos and books often go into much more detail about the issues involved which is helpful to some women. The cost of such material, however, can make it difficult to provide them in a clinic situation unless women are asked to pay a deposit to ensure their return. This then becomes an added administrative task to add to an already busy person's job, whoever it may be. It may be better to ask your local library to consider stocking books about the subject which you could then recommend.

Dedicated clinic

When there was additional funding available to practices for running specific clinics, menopause clinics were just one of the many clinics being held which were dedicated to a specific disease or client group. Asthma clinics, hypertension clinics, weight loss clinics, 'stop smoking' clinics and so on, became the norm for those practices large enough to warrant them and with the staff to run them. Whether or not one agreed with the way they were established or the financial arrangements behind them, there is no doubt that some people liked the idea that a clinic would be run by someone who was both interested and knowledgeable in the subject, with appointment times that reflected the consultations required and in a room or rooms which were conducive to the tests or investigations necessary (Roberts, 1996).

Aims

In deciding to establish a clinic, consider what you hope to achieve. Do you simply wish to make information more widely available or do you hope to reach specific women who would not otherwise attend? Is your long-term aim to reduce fractures and cardiovascular incidents or do you hope to help symptomatic women in the short term? Considering such issues will help you identify the best means to achieve these aims, in your situation. You will need to consider your own particular patient population – will daytime appointments be useful or do most women work? Will women feel safe attending the clinic in the dark evenings? Do you have a particular ethnic group whom you are hoping to inform – would you value an interpreter? Consider the literacy level of your likely group and tailor the literature accordingly.

If you decide to run a menopause clinic, you are implying to your patients that this is an issue which concerns you enough to try to improve the care that is given at this time. Women themselves seem to like clinics dedicated to issues such as menopause or family planning, but because they are not always cost-effective, many practices cannot afford to run them. This does not mean of course, that the treatment is any less effective when prescribed from a general clinic, or even that the staff are any less sympathetic, but reality being what it is, it does occasionally mean that time is too limited to give the care that is really needed. Holding a dedicated menopause clinic may mean that women will receive that little

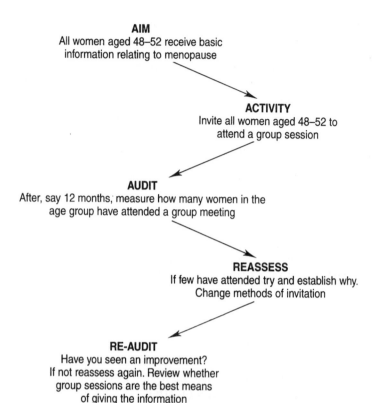

AIM
All women aged 48–52 receive basic
information relating to menopause

ACTIVITY
Invite all women aged 48–52 to
attend a group session

AUDIT
After, say 12 months, measure how many women in the
age group have attended a group meeting

REASSESS
If few have attended try and establish why.
Change methods of invitation

RE-AUDIT
Have you seen an improvement?
If not reassess again. Review whether
group sessions are the best means
of giving the information

Figure 9.5   Reassessing protocol following audit.

extra attention than if they are seen in a busy general clinic.

Benefits of a dedicated clinic are:

- Longer appointment times
- Sympathetic and knowledgeable staff
- Incorporates well women advice alongside specific menopause advice
- Counselling, assessing and monitoring all done in same clinic

Disadvantages of dedicated clinic are:

- Appointment times are fixed
- Patient loses her choice of doctor
- Work can be repetitive for staff

Audit

Audit is simply a means of measuring standard of care. Audit can be as simple or as complex as you choose, depending on what you are trying to measure and over what period of time. One reason for audit is to ensure that standards of care are being maintained, even when a variety of health professionals are involved. Aims or goals can be set, a protocol established to meet those aims and then an audit will help measure the effectiveness of the activity. As a result of an audit, you may choose to rethink your protocol in order to be more effective at reaching your stated goals or aims. An example is shown in Fig. 9.5.

In relation to menopause and HRT in primary care settings, you may consider an audit of the following:

- Number of hysterectomized women not on HRT
- Why women in your practice stop HRT
- How many women in your practice have continued on HRT for more than 5 years.
- Number of women who have had both ovaries removed but are not on HRT

Community pharmacists

Pharmacists have an important role to play in educating women about HRT and ensuring that they understand how to take their treatment. A woman may seek the advice of the community pharmacist about her HRT, particularly with regard to issues such as side-effects or practicalities of when or how to use the treatment. Therefore it is important that the pharmacists have accurate information to hand, otherwise it can lead to more confusion on the part of the client. Practice nurses and GPs can help the local pharmacists by keeping them informed of any new regimens which are commonly prescribed, particularly if they are 'tailor made' regimens.

QUESTIONS PATIENTS ASK*

Once you start to counsel women about menopause and hormone replacement therapy, you will soon find that they turn to you for help and advice about their treatment. They may not have fully understood how to use the HRT, or they may be experiencing difficulties once they are on it. It is helpful to encourage women to contact you if they do have anxieties or concerns as many minor problems can easily be solved through a telephone conversation, saving the need for a further appointment. If women are unable to get help about a particular problem, they are more likely to simply stop treatment of their own accord. Women may also be returning to you for regular monitoring. It is important that they feel able to express any concerns and that you try to resolve any problems they may have. If women are able to ask questions they will have more confidence in their HRT and also have a greater understanding of the treatment they have been prescribed.

Do I need HRT?

This is a difficult question to answer because the needs vary greatly between individuals. You should discuss a woman's symptoms and how much they are bothering her at present. What one woman might find intolerable, another will cope with more readily, depending on her lifestyle and work demands. It is also helpful to establish what the woman herself expects from HRT – is she realistic in considering the benefits? You should also discuss her risk of heart disease and osteoporosis, as this may be an influencing factor in her decision to take HRT.

After a frank discussion about her symptoms, risks for heart disease and osteoporosis, as well as a frank discussion about side-effects and risks of HRT, you will be in a better position to help her decide whether to try HRT.

---

*Some of these were first published in *Community Nurse* (1995) in an article by the author.

Do I need a blood test?

Women often believe that a blood test will help measure whether they need HRT or not. However, most women do not need a blood test as actual levels of circulating oestrogen do not directly correlate to severity of symptoms. Follicle stimulating hormone (FSH) levels fluctuate widely during the perimenopause, even whilst symptoms may be quite severe. Measuring FSH may be useful in women who have had a hysterectomy and are vital for the diagnosis of premature menopause, but in many other circumstances, patient history alone is sufficient for a diagnosis.

Will HRT help all my symptoms?

If an adequate dose of HRT is taken, symptoms caused by oestrogen deficiency will gradually disappear. Problems arise when a woman experiences symptoms which arise around the time of the menopause which may not be truly hormone-related. This may include symptoms such as tiredness, irritability, loss of libido and headaches. Whilst such symptoms may be caused by oestrogen deficiency, they may equally be caused by other influencing factors in a woman's life. It may be worth trying HRT, but you should advise a woman that HRT is not necessarily the answer.

What is the best form of HRT?

Women are becoming more aware of the different types of HRT – pills, patches, gels and implants – and may seek advice as to which one is the best. The secret is to choose a route with which the woman herself feels comfortable and to encourage her to persevere with this therapy for at least 3 months. Later, doses may need changing, progestogens may need adjusting, but ultimately the 'best' HRT is the one which suits the woman at that particular time. Both women themselves and health professionals need to be flexible enough to recognize that some treatments will suit some women more than others.

Aren't I just delaying the inevitable?

Taking HRT does not delay the menopause itself. It simply masks the fact that these hormonal changes are occurring. Women on HRT do not experience the menopause all over again when they stop HRT, although they may have a few symptoms if they do not stop HRT gradually. The menopause will occur whether or not HRT is taken, oestrogen simply makes the transition through the climacteric easier for some women.

How do I know the dose of HRT is right for me?

Women must feel confident that the HRT prescribed for them, is not only effective but also safe. If a woman is taking HRT for symptom relief, the right dose is that which controls her symptoms adequately, without too many side-effects. For those taking HRT for prevention of osteoporosis there is a standard dose of each preparation which is considered to be bone protective (see Chapter 3).

Can I safely take other medications alongside my HRT?

You can safely take other prescribed medications whilst using HRT, although you should advise your doctor that you are taking HRT. You can also take vitamins or dietary supplements if you wish.

Can I get pregnant on HRT?

Women who are truly postmenopausal can be reassured that even though they may see a return of bleeding, they are not fertile again. Women who start HRT whilst peri-menopausal could theoretically get pregnant, so are advised to continue using a contraceptive method alongside their HRT (see Chapter 5).

Can I adjust the dose of HRT I take, according to how I am feeling?

Fluctuations of oestrogen often cause symptoms. The aim of HRT is to achieve a steady level of oestrogen circu-

PATIENT SUPPORT
– Questions patients ask

lating in the body, whilst maintaining a safe effect on the body. It is therefore unhelpful to repeatedly change the amount of HRT you take. However you may find that the dose of oestrogen you require changes over the time that you take HRT. For example you may need a higher dose when you start and then a lower dose later on. You should discuss this with your doctor or practice nurse who will help you assess the dose you require. You should not change the dose on your own accord.

Could HRT be causing my headaches, rather than relieving them?

Headaches may occur as a menopause symptom, particularly in association with tiredness and poor sleep pattern. Headaches can also occur if the dose of oestrogen in HRT is not right for you. Some women experienc headaches as a side-effect of progestogen in cyclical HR'i'. Headaches can also be caused by many other factors, such as stress, anxiety or poor eyesight. If you continue to suffer headaches whilst on HRT, it may be worth trying a different type or dose, whilst also trying to establish whether there is another cause for them.

Can I simply stop HRT without causing any harm?

It is quite safe to simply stop HRT at the end of a cycle. However, you may experience mild symptoms again, as your body gets used to a lower oestrogen level. It therefore makes sense to stop the oestrogen gradually over a 2–3 month period. You can do this by taking the oestrogen on alternate days, or by changing patches less frequently than usual. Meanwhile if you have not had a hysterectomy, it is important that you continue taking the progestogen part of the regimen as normal until all oestrogen has been stopped. If you have had an implant, you may need to continue the progestogen for much longer, even if you are no longer having oestrogen implants (see Chapter 6).

I am going to have an operation, do I need to stop my HRT?

There is often no need to stop HRT prior to surgery. However, some surgeons and anaesthetists will advise that HRT is stopped 6 weeks prior to an operation. You should check well in advance or you could risk having your operation cancelled at the last moment.

I have been taking HRT for 9 weeks, but it does not seem to be working – shall I try a different one?

You should try to persevere with a particular HRT for at least 3 months before deciding that it does not suit you. Some women take longer than others to 'settle' on to a therapy. If after about 3 months on a particular HRT, you still feel that it is ineffective, return for further assessment. You may require an increase in dose, or a change of type of HRT.

I have been prescribed HRT, but when should I actually start it?

If you are still seeing periods, you should start your HRT near the beginning of a natural cycle, so that your bleeding remains regular in the early few months on HRT. If your periods have finished you can start you HRT as soon as you wish.

How soon can I expect to see an improvement in my symptoms?

Flushes and sweats often start to improve very quickly – even within a week or two of starting HRT. Other symptoms may take much longer to improve – some psychological symptoms may take months to improve. You can expect to see maximum benefit after you have been on treatment for about 3–4 months.

When should my bleed start and how long should it be?

If you are taking a cyclical form of HRT, your bleed should come towards the end of the progestogen phase of treatment, or shortly afterwards. If it regularly starts much earlier than this you may need a change of dose of progestogen. Most women on cyclical HRT experience between 4 and 7 days of bleeding, although it can be much shorter than this. Women using a continuous oestrogen/progestogen regimen may experience irregular bleeding for several months, eventually settling to no bleeding at all in most cases.

After several years on cyclical HRT, my bleeds have now stopped altogether – does this matter?

A small proportion of women on cyclical HRT do not bleed at all, even though they are taking the progestogen regularly. When a woman has been on HRT for many years, the endometrium can become atrophic, so no bleeding occurs. This is considered satisfactory, although an ultrasound scan may be performed to ensure that the womb lining is not thickened. If it does appear thickened, an endometrial biopsy may be performed to ensure that no unhealthy changes have occurred.

Can I delay my bleed so that the timing is more convenient, for example on holiday?

If you have been using HRT for some time, you can often change the timing of your bleed by adjusting the timing of the progestogen. It is best to do so gradually, over a couple of months before the one you wish to change, gradually delaying or bringing forward the progestogen so that the timing of the bleed changes. Alternatively you could try simply missing one month of progestogen to avoid a bleed. It should work, but you may see some occasional spotting instead of a regular bleed. It is not advisable to regularly miss out a course of progestogen because it is possible that the womb lining will build up and not be shed.

Does it matter if I take my HRT pills in the morning or at night?

For most women, it does not make any difference what time of day the tablets are taken. A few women experience mild nausea if they take tablets first thing in the morning, so prefer to take them later in the day or at night. It is important to try and take them at roughly the same time each day, whether it is morning or evening, simply to make them easier to remember.

What do I do if I miss a pill or a patch?

If you miss a pill, it is not worth trying to 'catch up' by taking two together next day. Simply leave the one you missed and continue with the regimen. If you miss a tablet during the progestogen phase, you may see some light bleeding a couple of days later. You should try not to miss too many pills because you may see a return of your symptoms within a short time. If you forget to change a patch, simply change it when you remember, then change it again on the day that it would normally be next due. It is most convenient if you always try to change your patch on the same day(s) of the week as this makes it easier to remember.

Can I sunbathe or use a sunbed whilst wearing a patch?

It is advised that the patch should be covered or removed whilst using a sunbed. Ordinary sunbathing should not affect the patch. If you have slight allergy to a patch, sunbathing may make it worse.

Can I swim and shower whilst using a patch?

Newer patches are designed to stay on whilst you swim or shower. You may find that older style reservoir patches may fall off in a prolonged hot bath. These patches can be dried and reapplied after the bath if necessary, although this may make them less effective.

Does it matter where I put the patch or gel?

Patches should be applied below the waistline, usually to the buttock or abdomen. Gel should be applied to the upper arms or inner thigh area. You should never apply a patch or gel to the breast area. It is common sense to avoid using the same area of skin all the time when changing your patches – change the site regularly and avoid applying a patch or gel to an area of broken skin.

CONCLUSION

Some would argue that all women from the ages of 45 years upwards should receive information about the menopause even if they do not actually ask for it. This may simply mean providing literature in the waiting room, or raising the subject when they are in the surgery for something else. The most appropriate time may be when she attends for her regular cervical smear test. A brief comment or question can ensure that the woman knows that discussion is invited if and when she wishes. The woman is then free to raise the issue again, or simply to leave it at this time. Some women may not realize that help is available, or may be too embarrassed to raise the issue specifically. All nurses should be providing information to women about menopause, whether it is ward nurses, family planning nurses, health visitors, occupational health nurses or others. In some situations it is the nurse who is likely to be more available for giving advice and it is vital that such opportunities are taken.

It is only as women feel able to ask the necessary questions and to have an open frank discussion that they can then make a decision which is right for them. In order to do this, they need information not just about menopause and what it is, or HRT, but also other health issues, lifestyle and nonhormonal therapies as well as an understanding of the changes which occur in a woman's body at this time.

REFERENCES

Amarant Trust National Survey (1992)

Beltchez P (1989) Hormone replacement therapy – deserves wider use. *Br. Med. J.* **298**: 1467.

Draper J & Roland M (1990) Perimenopausal women's views on taking HRT to prevent osteoporosis. *Br. Med. J.* **300**: 786–788.

Garnett T, Mitchell A & Studd J (1991) Patterns of referral to a menopause clinic. *J. R. Soc. Med.*. **84**: 128.

Hope S & Rees MCP (1995) Why do British women start and stop HRT? *J. Br. Menopause Soc.*

National Opinion Poll Survey (1991) The menopause revolution – how far have we come? Giba Geigy: Horsham.

Roberts PJ (1991) The menopause and HRT – Views of women in general practice receiving HRT. *Br. J. Gen. Practice* **41**: 421–424.

Roberts PJ (1996) Comparison of care between a General Practice Clinic and General Surgeries: The views of women using HRT. *J. Br. Menopause Soc.* **2**: 1.

Rothert M, Rovner D, Holmes M et al (1990) Women's use of information regarding HRT. *Res. Nurs. Health* **13**: 355–366.

Shine U (1995) The true facts on HRT. *Practice Nurse* 1 Dec.: 528–529.

Sinclair HK, Bond CM, Taylor RJ (1993) HRT: A study of women's knowledge and attitudes. *Br. J. Gen. Practice* **43**: 365–370.

Appendix

Resources

SUGGESTED BOOKS

For the nonmedical reader

Books that cover many aspects of the menopause, including HRT in some depth:

Menopause by Miriam Stoppard, Dorling Kindersley Ltd 1994

Understanding HRT and the menopause, by Dr Robert CD Wilson. Consumer's Association 1995 (2nd edn)

Menopause and HRT, by Heather Kirby (in association with Marie Stopes Clinic), Ward Lock 1994

Books specifically about osteoporosis:

Understanding Osteoporosis, by Wendy Cooper, Arrow Books 1990

More detailed books about HRT:

Hormone Replacement Therapy – your guide to making an informed choice, by Rosemary Nicol. Vermillion 1993

HRT – Making your own decision, by Patsy Westcott. Thorsons 1993

Books describing a personal experience through the menopause transition – including some humorous moments:

The silent passage, by Gail Sheehy. Harper Collins 1993

It is hot in here or is it me? by Gayle Sand, Bloomsbury Publishing 1993

Books written from an holistic approach, with an emphasis on natural or alternative treatments:

Menopause – a practical self help guide for women, by Raewyn Mackenzie. Sheldon Press 1994

All about the menopause and its treatment without drugs, by David Potterton. Foulsham 1995

A Change for the better – a woman's guide through the menopause, by Patricia Davis. The CW Daniel Company Ltd 1993

Beat the menopause without HRT, by Maryon Stewart. Headline Book Publishing 1995

The Pause – Positive Approaches to Menopause, by Lonnie Barbach. Bantam Books 1994

Aimed at health professionals

Menopause and Osteoporosis Therapy Manual for GPs and Practice Nurses, available from National Osteoporosis Society

Hormone replacement therapy – your questions answered, by Malcolm Whitehead and Val Godfree. Churchill Livingstone 1992

Osteoporosis – A clinical guide, by Anthony D Woolf and Allan St John Dixon. Martin Dinitz 1990

Osteoporosis, by John A Kanis. Blackwell Science 1995

VIDEOS

These videos are aimed at lay women and are generally around 20–30 minutes in length. They each deal with the subject in different ways and you are advised to see the video before recommending it! Some are distributed by pharmaceutical companies and have a strong emphasis on the need for HRT.

The Good HRT Guide – presented by Margi Clarke (Good Sex Guide). Information about HRT is provided in a lighthearted manner. Gynaecologist John Studd provides the medical input. Distributed by Rhone Poulence Rorer (pharmaceutical company).

You, the Menopause and HRT – TV Doctor Mark Porter answers questions commonly asked about menopause and HRT. He is joined by Angela Buckingham (a patient) describing her experiences of the menopause. Distributed by Ciba Pharmaceuticals.

How to live through the menopause – Sunday Times - Your health in your hands Series 1991. An overview of what happens at the time of menopause and informative discussion about HRT.

What you really need to know about HRT. A formal presentation of the facts about the menopause and HRT. Presented by Dr Robert Buckman and introduced by John Cleese. Sponsored by Schering Healthcare.

USEFUL ADDRESSES

If you require more information about issues discussed in this book, you may wish to contact one or more of the following. Please remember to enclose a stamped addressed envelope with your enquiry.

British Menopause Society
36 West St
Marlow
Bucks
SL7 2NB

Multidisciplinary professional organization for those health professionals working in the field of menopause. At present the BMS does not have facilities for enquiries from the lay public.

National Osteoporosis Society
PO Box 10
Radstock
Bath
BA3 3YB

Provides excellent literature for both lay and health professionals at reasonable cost, on many issues relating to osteoporosis. Helpline available.

Women's Health Information Service
52–54 Featherstone St
London
EC1Y 8RT

Information available for lay women on many health-related issues.

The Amarant Trust
11–13 Charterhouse Buildings
London
EC1M 7AN

Information available about menopause related issues, mainly for lay women. Recorded helplines available.

Family Planning Association
2–12 Pentonville Road
London
N1 9FP

For information on any issue relating to reproductive and sexual health, for both lay and health professionals. Helpline available for issues relating to contraception only.

Women's Nutritional Advisory Service
PO Box 268
Lewes
East Sussex
BN7 2QN

Offers specific dietary, nutritional and exercise advice for women with premenstrual syndrome or going through the menopause.

Women's Health Concern
PO Box 1629
London
W8 6AU

Literature available on all aspects of women's health. Helpline available.

Relate
Head Office
Little Church St
Rugby
CV21 3AP

Alternative therapies

British Homeopathic Association
27a Devonshire St
London
W1N 1RJ

Complementary Therapies in Nursing, Special Interest
Group
The Royal College of Nursing
20 Cavendish Square
London
W1M 0AB

Faculty of Herbal Medicine
(General Council and Register of Consultant Herbalists)
Grosvenor House
40 Sea Way
Middleton on Sea
West Sussex
PA22 7AA

Register of Qualified Aromatherapists
54a Gloucester Ave
London
NW1 8JD

British Acupuncture Association and Register
34 Alderney St
London
SW1V 4EU

Index

Page numbers in *italic* refer to illustrations and tables; **bold** page numbers indicate main discussions.